ESSAYS THAT WILL GET YOU INTO

PHYSICIAN
ASSISTANT
SCHOOL

Andrew J. Rodican, PA-C

ISBN:1481129759
ISBN 13:9781481129756
Library of Congress Control Number: 2012922897
CreateSpace Independent Publishing Platform
North Charleston, South Carolina

Table of Contents

Part II: Writing

Preface

Sometimes, even the best candidates don't get into the physician assistant school of their choice because they don't know how to write a strong admissions essays. That is why I wrote this book. I don't want that to happen to you.

Several years ago, I was a member of the Physician Assistant Program Admissions Committee at Yale University. While on that committee, I discovered that there are certain principles and practices that top applicants use to make themselves very appealing to an admissions committee. I've spent 15 years refining those practices and principles and assisting those who wish to enter the profession get into the school of their choice. I've used my gifts as a mentor and teacher to lend a hand to others and I want to help you in this book.

I graduated from the Yale University School of Medicine Physician Associate (PA) Program in 1994. I have been a practicing PA for over 16 years and am the founder and Associate Medical Director of Medical Weight Loss Centers in East Haven, CT (www.MedWeightLossCenters.com.) I am also the founder of AJR Associates (www.AndrewRodican.com), which is a consulting firm dedicated to helping Physician Assistant school applicants get accepted to PA school.

In addition to this book, I've published two other books designed to help PA school applicants achieve success in getting into PA school. In my first book, *The Ultimate Guide to Getting Into Physician Assistant School*, now in the 3rd edition (McGraw-Hill Medical, 2010), I outline the entire application process and give readers general information about PA programs. *How To "Ace" The Physician Assistant School Interview*, *The Ultimate Guide to Getting Into Physician Assistant School* (AJR Associates, 2011) is my second book. It focuses exclusively on the PA school interview. I encourage you to read those books as well as they contain much helpful information.

This book is separated into two parts: preparation and writing. While you could read the entire book in one sitting, I recommend you take some time to process the information. You will want to contemplate your writing preferences and needs before you start writing and you'll want to let your ideas gel while you are writing. And be sure to give yourself plenty of time to read and process the material. Don't wait until a week before your essay is due to read the book. Read it early and then re-read the helpful sections as you write.

I hope you enjoy and appreciate the suggestions in this book. And remember that more information and help can be found at www.AndrewRodican.com.

Best of luck as you continue to pursue your dream to be a Physician Assistant.

Andrew J. Rodican, PA-C

Introduction

WHY THE ESSAY MATTERS

In 2012, the US Bureau of Labor Statistics predicted that jobs in the Physician Assistant (PA) profession would increase 30 percent between 2010 and 2020. This is a much greater growth rate than the national average of 14 percent for overall projected job growth.

Since you are reading this book, you are most likely considering a career as a Physician Assistant. And given the above statistic, you have made a good choice, right?

Right. However, competition for getting accepted into PA school is increasing because others have also heard about the positives of being a PA. While we'd all like to think the individuals who get accepted are the best applicants, this is not necessarily the case. Those who get accepted are the ones who have been thoughtful and attentive to the application process.

Even if you meet or exceed all of the prerequisites, you need to write a great essay to be invited to an interview. The essay is your opportunity to distinguish yourself from the other candidates and convince the admissions committee that they should invite you in for an interview.

You want to write an amazing essay—one that will significantly increase your chances of getting invited to interview at the PA school(s) of your choice. This book will help you write that winning essay.

But before we get to the details of how to write a great essay, you will need a little context on the profession and a bit more information about the process so that you can accomplish your goal: a spot in the PA program of your choice!

OVERVIEW OF THE FIELD

The Physician Assistant profession dates back to the 1960s, when there was a shortage and uneven geographic distribution of primary-care physicians in the United States. In an attempt to ease the problems associated with this shortage, Dr. Eugene Stead of Duke University Medical Center decided to start a Physician Assistant training program and assembled an inaugural class. This class was composed of former US Navy hospital corpsman and US Army combat medics, who had received considerable medical training during their military service.

This class graduated on October 6, 1967, a date that is now considered to be the official anniversary of the PA profession. October 6 through 11 has been designated as National Physician Assistant Week in honor of this class.

During the 1970s, the US Army was the primary user of physician assistants. The army was losing many physicians to civilian practice, and they quickly saw the benefit of PAs. In 1971, Congress authorized the training of four hundred army PAs. The first army class graduated in July 1973. The other services quickly followed the army's lead and established their own PA programs.

From that first class of four PAs at Duke University Medical Center, the PA profession has grown to over 88,000 PAs currently eligible to practice. It is projected that there will be demand for 150,000 physician assistants by the year 2020. And it is likely that the demand will continue to grow long after 2020.

WHO THEY ARE AND WHAT THEY PRACTICE

Just over 65 percent of practicing physician assistants are female. The average age for a PA student is twenty-seven. Practice options are varied, and PAs may practice in many areas including primary care, surgical specialties, emergency medicine, internal medicine, pediatrics, and other specialty areas. Physician Assistants can work for others (in clinics and hospitals) or even for themselves (private practice with other health-care professionals working for them).

THE FIVE MAJOR MISTAKES IN PA SCHOOL CONSIDERATION

Before you apply, it is important to consider the ramifications of going to PA school. I have found that there are five major mistakes made by candidates as they consider school or while they are in school.

Mistake No. 1: Financial Fears

Physician assistant school is expensive. It is also a lot of work and requires time spent studying and in clinical rotations. Candidates are often unsure whether or not to quit a current job. While careful consideration is important, you shouldn't let financial fears get in the way of making the best decisions for you.

Most programs display costs for PA school on their website, but you can expect to spend over thirty thousand dollars per year on school. PAs earn anywhere between $70,000 (usually the upper seventies) and $110,000 per year. From these numbers, you can calculate your return on investment (i.e., two years of tuition costs with no salary compared to your earning potential when you get out).

Additionally, ask yourself the following questions:

1.   Can I afford to become a PA?
2.   Can I afford not to become a PA?
3.   Where will I be in five years (as a PA or not)?
4.   Can I afford to give up my current job while I attend school?
5.   Is my current employment secure?

Answering these questions honestly will provide you with the insight you need to make the best decisions for you and your family and to avoid making a mistake related to financial fears.

Mistake No. 2: Mistaken Motivations

Passion is the rocket fuel that drives the car to success. In order to sacrifice what is needed to be successful in physician assistant school and to work as a physician assistant, you will need to be sure that you want to be a PA. If you are both serious about becoming a PA and are passionate and committed to becoming a PA, you will be successful. Without both, you are just another used Chevy on the lot.

Passion comes from the Latin word meaning "to suffer." In other words, to become a PA, you must be willing to sacrifice in order to achieve your goal. To be willing to suffer, you must be motivated and have a clear goal.

Researchers who have studied successful people have determined that they accomplished their goals by doing three things. First, they wrote their goals on paper. The mere act of writing them out—articulating them on paper—reinforced the goal. Second, they held themselves accountable for their goals. Finally, they made a commitment to themselves and others to accomplish those goals.

Mistake No. 3: Application Blunders

The single biggest mistake applicants make during the application process is not paying strict enough attention to the details. Being successful as a PA requires attention to detail because you are dealing with patients' health. A careless mistake can make the difference between health and illness and in the most serious cases, life and death.

Mistakes like not following directions or making careless typos and grammatical errors will communicate to the committee that you don't attend to details. A careless application means a careless professional.

Recommendations can also cause problems in the application process. When thinking about recommendations, you need to consider many things.

First, applicants often assume that a letter of recommendation from a prestigious physician or scholar improves their chances of being accepted into PA school. That is not necessarily true, especially if that person doesn't know you well—which is often the case. You are far better off getting a letter from someone who knows you well and can speak about you from personal experience. These people can give specific examples of why they think you will be a good candidate for PA school and the profession, which makes for a stronger and "truer" recommendation.

Second, many recommenders write as if the applicant is applying for a job, which you are not. They should focus on you as a potential student, not employee. Also consider this when you select your recommender. A person who can recommend you for a job may not be the same person you would like to have recommend you for PA school.

Third, remember that your letter is not a character reference. Someone you know from church or your grandmother who has had a lot of medical care can attest to your many good qualities but will not be very helpful at assessing your candidacy to PA school.

Finally, try to pick someone who can be as unbiased as possible. If the chair of surgery in a large medical center in your hometown is a friend of the family and knows you well, he or she may still not be a good reference if the committee believes that he or she is unable to be objective about you.

It's a tricky balance to achieve and requires that you give this part of your application some time and good thought.

Mistake No. 4: Getting all the way to the interview and missing the mark

If you are successful with your application and essay, you will be invited to an interview. As was mentioned earlier, preparation is key. There are some key things to think about regarding the interview, and applicants often fail to take this important step.

You need to know about current "hot" topics, such as health-care reform, managed care, and the role of the PA in the future. Familiarize yourself with the laws and limitations of PAs in the state in which you are interviewing, as well as your "home" state. You must also know who will be conducting the interview, whether you will have an individual, group, or casual round-table interview, and how to handle those dynamics. You need to know the scoring criteria, and finally—and most important—you must know answers to the questions the interviewer(s) will ask!

Mistake No. 5: Essay Pitfalls

This is important: Applicants who fail to use the personal statement to create a frame for their candidacy are making a serious mistake.

Your personal statement may be the single most important piece of writing you will do in your medical career. Do not use this valuable real estate to reiterate the contents of your résumé. Use this statement to make a personal connection with the readers and create a desire in them to meet you in person.

The essay is your ticket to the interview; however, it can also be the kiss of death if it's not well done!

Presentation is important. Badly written essays give a negative impression and may even alienate the admissions officers who read them. Essays are the most time-consuming part of the admissions process for the admissions officers, and reading a poorly written essay can be a painful experience for them. If they feel pain reading your essay, you will not be invited in for an interview.

In this book, you will learn the details of how to write an effective essay. The book is divided into several chapters with each chapter focusing on important features of the essay.

PART I
Preparation

Thinking Strategically

1

UNDERSTANDING THE WRITING PROCESS

One common misunderstanding about good writing is that it is the result of moments of inspiration. While these moments can be helpful, good writing is not the result of inspiration—rather, it is the result of hard work and numerous rewrites. So before you start, know that this essay will take some time

Further, the best writing doesn't just "happen" when you sit down. Good writing requires preparation and then *multiple* drafts. Be prepared to work through several drafts and sit through many writing sessions.

Preparation for good writing also requires forethought. Think about what you want to say as well as how you want to say it; let an idea "roll around" in your mind a bit and then try committing it to paper. Being strategic about writing can improve your chances of creating a winning essay.

This chapter provides an overview of strategies that will prepare you to write. I offer you commonsense, yet also very important, help to get you on the right track with writing your PA school essay.

WHERE TO WRITE

Some people need a quiet room with a desk. Others prefer a noisy coffee shop. According to a *Chicago Tribune* article entitled Where Writers Write, many famous writers have very specific requirements about their most inspirational places to put pen to paper. Oscar Hijuelos (*The Mambo Kings Play Songs of Love*) needs a quiet, private space preferably with a view. Jodi Picoult (author of numerous fiction novels) writes in her attic office. Tayari

Jones (*Silver Sparrow*) writes in the spare bedroom in her apartment. And Wally Lamb (*She's Come Undone*) prefers his finished basement for writing.[1]

While you aren't writing a novel, you still need to consider where you do your best thinking and writing and try to work in that setting each and every time you write. Your mind will automatically shift into writing mode if you follow a routine related to where and when you write. While this may seem like an unnecessary step in the writing process, remember that your PA essay has the potential to change the trajectory of your life, so spending a bit of time to think about space can be an important part of your process.

WHEN TO WRITE

It is also important to think about when you should write. Some people like to write early in the morning when they feel fresh. Others like to write late at night.

Don't plan to write at a time when your creative brain has shut down (writing is a creative process after all) or after you have just completed an intense mental task (e.g., a test). Think about when you do your best writing, and plan to work on your essay during that time.

STIMULATING THE WRITING BRAIN

It's happened to all of us. You sit down with a pen and paper or at your computer and…nothing. You don't know how to start, and nothing is coming from your blocked brain.

Never fear, even great writers need stimulation at times. Are you someone for whom reading stimulates your desire to write? Or does journaling get your creative juices flowing? Or maybe you find quiet meditation gets you into the writing mood. Having a writing routine will help you when you get to writing your essay.

Here are some fun exercises to get your mind ready to write:

1. Write down fifty adjectives to describe yourself.
2. Write a paragraph or two about your life five years from now when you are a successful PA. What do you like about your job? What do you enjoy about being with patients? What do you like about the practice of medicine?

---

1   Alexia Elejalde-Ruiz, *Chicago Tribune*, June 24, 2011,
http://articles.chicagotribune.com/2011-06-24/entertainment/
ct-books-0625-where-writers-write-20110624_1_authors-novel-attic.

3. Write a fictional story about a PA hero or heroine. What would he or she do? Who are this PA's patients? What do these patients think of your hero or heroine?
4. Talk aloud (to yourself or a friend) about what you want to say in your essay or how you might start it. If you are a very verbal person, this can be a great way to get your writing brain engaged.
5. Write one sentence each about five people you admire and what you admire about them.

These are just a few examples of ways to get warmed up for writing. Just like in physical exercise, warm-ups can be helpful. The Internet is filled with suggestions for writing warm-ups, so if none of these ideas inspire you and you are still not sure how to start, check online.

SCHEDULING AND DEADLINES

Remember also to put yourself on a *schedule*. Create a time line that includes deadlines for making an outline, completing a first draft, doing revisions, and finally finishing the essay. Allow yourself adequate time for all creative processes as well as revisions and edits. Often starting at the end (the deadline) and working backward with your schedule will allow you to see the quantity of time you will need to dedicate to this task.

While deadlines can be hard for some of us, they provide the structure for you to keep organized. Remember to include in your schedule flexibility for personal or family emergencies, other work deadlines or commitments, computer problems, et cetera. The last thing you want to be in a position to have to do is request an extension on your application—even if it is a legitimate issue or problem.

MANAGING WRITER'S BLOCK

Finally, prepare for *writer's block*. Even professional writers get stumped at times. If your writing gets stalled, it is probably your brain telling you it is time for a break—so take one.

Do free writing (more on that in the next section), exercise, go for a walk, or get a cup of coffee or tea. In sum, distracting yourself for a minute or ten can assist you in giving the writing part of your brain enough of a break that it is fresh and ready to start again when you return.

PROCRASTINATION

Everyone procrastinates at times, and students have been known to procrastinate more than others. Rather than work, we surf the Internet, clean our closets, go on social media sites, eat, et cetera. While we all procrastinate at times, it is estimated that 20 percent of all people are chronic procrastinators. If you are one of those people, there is hope, but you will need to be disciplined.

Here are some tips:

1. Estimate correctly. Some of us procrastinate because we've underestimated how long it takes to do something—and we know it. If you see a trend, adapt. In other words, if tasks usually take two times longer than you expect, schedule a task to take two times longer.
2. Make a list, and set a schedule.
3. Set realistic goals. As I have mentioned and will mention again later in this book, your essay will not be effective if you sit and write it in one session. So, be realistic about what you can do.
4. Promise yourself a reward when you complete your tasks. Sometimes a nice reward is all the motivation one needs to get moving.
5. Repeat the mantra: "Just do it now!"

Chapter 1 Checklist

- I have identified a specific location from which I can do my best writing.
- I have identified the best time of day for writing.
- I know several strategies for stimulating my brain to write.
- I have developed a schedule for completing my application essay.
- I have created deadlines for completion of parts of my essay and proofing and editing.
- I know what to do to move beyond writer's block.
- I know what to do when I am procrastinating to move myself to action.

Analyzing Your Audience

2

FINDING THE BEST FIT

Before you start writing your essay, you need to decide to which schools you wish to apply. With over 150 PA programs in the United States, there are many things to consider when you look at a program. The following questions are important to ask:

- Are there any discrepancies with the program's first-time pass/fail rates on the NCCPA boards, if applicable?
- What is the philosophy/focus of the program?
- What is the availability of clinical rotation sites?
- How is the quality of clinical rotation sites?
- Is there a cadaver lab?
- Who teaches the classes?
- What is the class size?

After you've found the schools to which you want to apply, you can begin your application letter. But first, you must think about your readers.

YOUR READERS

One of the most important preparation stages for writing your essay is to analyze your audience.

It is important to understand the review committee and its makeup. The admissions committee is made up of a combination of full-time admissions staff, faculty, maybe students, and possibly members of the community who practice in the field.

Think about what these individuals want, need, and expect as you create your essay. Communication models tell us that communication occurs only when what we intend for the reader to understand is indeed what the reader understands. So, taking some time to analyze your audience will help you be an effective communicator.

There are several basic aspects of your audience's background that you should consider. These include:

1. Their educational level. In your case, your readers will be highly educated.
2. Their professional experience. Your audience is made of admissions committee members and faculty, but they also have health-care experience and experience working with students so they know who is most likely to succeed in their program.
3. Their job responsibility. They have the responsibility of picking the best students for their program. So in addition to looking at background, test scores, and grades, they will also be looking for a good fit.
4. Their personal characteristics. This is harder to determine because you don't know the members of the admissions committee. However, you can do some research online and find out more about faculty interests and the values of the program (more on that later).
5. Your readers' cultural characteristics. You might not be able to determine much about culture, but you do have a rough idea of interests (health care) and background (educated). Work on being sensitive to culture and take care not to offend anyone with insensitive comments about culture, background, gender, sexual orientation, et cetera.

Giving some thought to the above issues will help you visualize your audience as you are writing. Doing so can be helpful for the essay's construction. It would be beneficial to talk with a PA you've met or know, as well as anyone in the health-care field who works with PAs, to have a better feel for what their working relationships—and therefore expectations—are. You can then incorporate that into your "knowing your audience" information.

And remember that admissions officers and committee members may look at many, many essays in a day. According to the Duke University website, 171 applications were submitted. You should hope that your essay is read early in the day. However, *prepare it as if it will be read at the end of the day!* In other words, don't waste the committee's time with a poorly crafted essay.

READERS' ATTITUDES AND EXPECTATIONS

You may not think you can analyze the attitudes and expectations of an admissions committee, but common sense can tell us a lot.

First, think about the readers' attitudes toward you. You are seeking admission to their program. They will most likely view you with a mix of curiosity, interest, and skepticism. The curiosity and interest come from their desire to get a well-qualified candidate for their program. And writing a good essay can pique that curiosity and interest (more on that in upcoming chapters). But they will also look at you with some skepticism because they know that most potential candidates paint a picture of themselves with only the best colors (as you should). This means then that you should be honest and careful that your essay reflects the "real" you. You will want to find a healthy mix of humility within the context of self-promotion.

Second, realize that these individuals are passionate about the PA field. Admissions committees are made up of individuals who care a good deal about what they are doing, and they will want to see that in a candidate as well. Be careful, however, that the enthusiasm you portray in the essay is genuine. Faux passion is very detectable.

Third, think about what values are important to the program. The following is taken from the Duke University Physician's Assistant Program website:

The Physician Assistant (PA) profession originated at Duke in the mid 1960s. Dr. Eugene A. Stead Jr., then Chairman of the Department of Medicine, believed that mid-level practitioners could increase consumer access to health services by extending the time and skills of the physician. Today, physician assistants are well-recognized and highly sought-after members of the health care team. Working interdependently with physicians, PAs provide diagnostic and therapeutic patient care in virtually all medical specialties and settings. They take patient histories, perform physical examinations, order laboratory and diagnostic studies and develop patient treatment plans. In all states, including North Carolina, PAs have the authority to write prescriptions. Their job descriptions are as diverse as those of their supervising physicians, and include patient education, team leadership, medical education, health administration and research.

PAs are interdependent members of the health care team. Many tasks have been integrated into the PA role, particularly in the institutional and larger clinic setting. While not always clinical in nature, these tasks are essential to the practice of the PA's supervising physician. For example, PAs in the tertiary care setting are often involved in the acquisition, recording and analysis of research data, the development of patient and public education programs, and the administration of their departments' clinical and educational services. Involvement in these other services has provided job advancement for PAs in these settings.[2]

---

2   Duke University Health System Physician Assistant Program, 2012, http://paprogram.mc.duke.edu/PA-Program/.

Note that the notion of being an interdependent member of a health care team is mentioned twice in the program description. Also of note is the fact that PAs must be able to perform many tasks and that the field itself is open to many options for practice.

The vision and mission of the program can also be helpful in thinking about how to approach the admissions committee in the essay. For example, here is the mission of the George Washington University Physician Assistant Program:

The GW Physician Assistant Program educates Physician Assistant students to practice evidence-based medicine, advocate for patients, and serve their communities.[3]

Clearly, GW has as a mission evidence-based medicine, but it also has a commitment to community service and patient advocacy. A well-written essay will speak to those aspects of their program.

In addition to values that may be idiosyncratic to a program, all programs will look for your motivation to be a PA. They will also be assessing your writing skills. They will be trying to understand the "real" you and discern your soft skills as well. I talk more about this in the next chapter.

In the next chapter, I also discuss more about analyzing the program, but this initial overview gives you some clues as to what is valued and thus some ways to frame your essay.

Chapter 2 Checklist

- I understand my audience's education level and know how this will affect my writing of the essay.
- I have determined which programs are the best fit for my interests and goals.
- I understand my audience's career backgrounds and experiences and know how this will affect my writing of the essay.
- I have been careful to be sensitive to cultural differences in my essay.
- I understand the overall values of the program to which I am applying.
- I understand how to create passion in my essay.
- I know how to create a healthy balance of self-promotion and humility in my essay.
- I know how to make my essay interesting and well organized for someone who might be reading it in the late afternoon on a Friday.

---

3   George Washington University, 2012, http://www.gwumc.edu/healthsci/academics/phyassist.cfm.

Defining Goals, Gathering Materials and Developing a Strategy

3

Before you start writing, you need to define your goals, gather your materials, and develop a strategy. I'll address these issues in this chapter and also give you some excerpts from sample essays (It is important to note that these essays are original and in some cases include errors which have not been edited for the purposes of this book).

DEFINE YOUR GOALS

Obviously, your primary objective is to present yourself strongly enough to get invited to interview at the PA school of your choice. But what do you want to communicate about yourself and your values that will convince the admissions committee to invite you to that interview?

Start with some questions: What are your dreams? If you could have any career right now, what would it be? Where do you see yourself in five years? Ten years? What kind of balance do you see in your life—work/family/helping others/hobbies, et cetera?

Now the critical question: is being a PA consistent with your life goals and your values? If yes, read on. If no, reassess.

There are two reasons why this step is important. First, this process (applying to and going through PA school) will not be easy; if you aren't truly committed to it, you should reassess to determine if it is really what you want. Second, while the admissions committee might not be able to see a conflict in your essay, they will be able to see if there is a conflict between your life goals and your career goals in the interview. So, you should be very certain they are aligned *before* that interview and even before you write the essay.

Now step back and look at what you have written. Do you see reoccurring themes? If so, what are they? I talk more about themes and the ways in which you can integrate them into the essay later in this chapter.

Before you start writing, you have a little more research to do.

DO YOUR RESEARCH ON THE PROFESSION

The admissions committee will expect you to have a thorough understanding of the PA profession and their school. Here are some questions you should be prepared to answer:

- What are some of the issues facing PAs today?
- How will health-care reform affect PAs?
- What are some of the greatest challenges facing PAs today?
- What is the difference between a PA and a nurse practitioner?
- Why don't you want to become a nurse practitioner?
- Why do you want to attend the programs to which you are applying?
- What do you know about the history of the programs to which you are applying?

You can find the answers to most of these questions in my book, *The Ultimate Guide to Getting into Physician Assistant School*[4] or on my website, www.AndrewRodican.com. However, there are many other resources available to you:

- American Academy of Physician Assistants (AAPA) (www.aapa.org)
- Student Academy of the American Academy of Physician Assistants (SAAPA) (http://www.aapa.org/student-academy)
- Physician Assistant Education Association (PAEA) (http://www.paeaonline.org)
- PA Programs Directory (http://www.paeaonline.org)
- Each PA Program's website
- PA students
- PA Forum (www.physicianassistantforum.com)
- Physician Assistants in the community

---

4   McGraw-Hill, 3rd ed. (2010).

Be sure to research the faculty at each PA program to which you receive an invitation to interview. Find out where they went to PA school, what area of medicine they practice, and what their relationship is to the PA program.

ASSESS THE SCHOOL

There are a variety of reasons why you may decide to apply to a particular school. It may be because the school has a good reputation. It may be because the school is located close to where you currently live. Or it may be because you appreciate the mission, vision, or values of the program. Whatever your reasons, it is important that your goals fit with the program to which you are applying.

With the Internet, it is fairly easy to assess a school. A visit to its website will tell you a lot about the values and mission of the program and also about the application process. Be aware that the website will tell you what they want you to know. You should also check ranking information and articles, which often include student comments about a program.

Now, let's look at a few programs to see how they vary.

Augsburg College is located in Minneapolis, Minnesota, and has a small class—admitting only thirty students per year. Their website describes the program in the following way:

Augsburg's Department of Physician Assistant Studies educates generalist physician assistants oriented toward service to underserved populations, both in rural and urban settings. The program includes full-time study in classes and clinical training. We are proud to say that all of our graduates are nationally board certified, and since the program's inception, our students have attained some of the highest mean scores on the national certifying examination administered by the National Commission on Certification of Physician Assistants (NCCPA).[5]

If you want to work in a suburban hospital with a mission to serve wealthier, insured patients or if you are interested in a very specific specialty, this program would not be a good fit for you.

The University of Wisconsin-Madison has two options for the PA program: a two-year in-person program and a three-year distance education program. Their mission, vision, and diversity statement communicate a lot about the program and potential fit:

---

5   Augsburg College, 2012, http://www.augsburg.edu/pa/.

Our Mission.

The mission of the University of Wisconsin-Madison Physician Assistant Program is to educate professionals committed to the delivery of comprehensive health care in a culturally and ethnically sensitive manner, with an emphasis on primary health care for populations and regions in need.

Our Vision.

The Program will serve as an academic and professional leader in the physician assistant profession by contributing its strengths in education, distance education, evidence-based practice, public health, community-based training and grant initiatives.

PA Program Diversity Statement

Diversity is central to the mission of the University of Wisconsin School of Medicine and Public Health and to the UW-Madison PA Program in meeting the health needs of the people of Wisconsin and beyond through excellence in education, research, patient care, and service. The UW-Madison PA Program puts specific emphasis on educating professionals committed to the delivery of comprehensive health care in a culturally and ethnically sensitive manner, with an emphasis on primary health care for populations and regions in need. To achieve this vision, the UW-Madison PA Program will recruit, admit and graduate a diverse student body, maintain an open, inclusive and respectful learning environment, and employ a curriculum that embraces individual differences and enhances cultural awareness. [6]

An applicant with a unique cultural background would have an advantage in a program like this, which is specifically looking for individuals who are culturally sensitive and who are interested in delivering "primary health care for populations and regions in need."

The last program we will examine is one that has a special focus. The University of Toledo admits around forty students per year but has a very specific focus:

The University of Toledo Department of Physician Assistant (PA) Studies was recently awarded a federal grant worth over $1,000,000! The grant is provided through the US Health and Human Services Health Resources and Services

---

[6]   Board of Regents of the University of Wisconsin, 2010, http://www.fammed.wisc.edu/pa-program/overview.

Administration (HRSA). As a result, the class size has increased to roughly 40 students. A new primary care specialty track has been created to use funding from the grant to provide $44,000 to five new, incoming PA students each year through 2015.

The University of Toledo Physician Assistant Program is the proud recipient of the 2011 Physician Assistant Education Association (PAEA) **Excellence Through Diversity Award** in recognition of outstanding achievements in fostering diversity in PA education through outreach and advocacy.[7]

This program would be great for someone with a diverse background and an interest in primary care.

We've reviewed only three of the nearly 150 PA programs out there, but even in these three, you can see vast differences. Failure to assess the program or failure to find a program that is a good fit for you will be a strike against you before you even start the application process. In other words, do your homework on the program and the fit through your self-assessment.

ASSESS YOURSELF

Knowing your strengths and weaknesses will be very important as you write your essay and also when you are interviewing with a program. So, it is critical that you assess yourself!

PA program admissions committees consider many factors in selection. First, cognitive ability is important. In other words, can you solve a problem? Can you articulate ideas logically and clearly? Are you perceptive? Are you organized? Do you have good time management skills, and do you understand how intense a PA program and practice is?

The admissions committee also seeks to assess the motivation of the candidate. They will wonder if you are strongly motivated or just testing the water. They will also want to know if being a PA is a backup for something else (e.g., medical school). They will examine your past schooling to determine if you have completed prerequisites and will assess your prior medical experiences.

They will also look at your knowledge of the profession. Do you seem to understand what being a PA entails? What is your attitude toward nurses and other members of the health-care team? Have you ever worked with any PAs? And do you know the history of the profession? Do you know the expectations of the profession?

They will also want to assess your interpersonal skills. Teaming is important in this profession, so they will want to determine if you can collaborate. They will wonder

7   University of Toledo, 2012, http://www.utoledo.edu/med/grad/pa/.

if you are empathic and compassionate. They will want to know if you get along well with others.

The committee will seek to determine if you can handle stress well. They will find out some of this at the interview (when you are under stress), but stories in the essay can also tell about stressful situations you handled with ease. They will also want to know if you can think on your feet.

Finally, they will want to get to know you as a person. Are you thoughtful and innovative? Are you mature? Are you driven? Do you have passion, and can you motivate others? There are many other positive personal characteristics that may be unique to you, and you will want to keep those in mind as you write your essay.

IDENTIFY YOUR THEMES

Now is the time to get specific in thinking about what you would bring to the profession as a PA. I present some essay excerpts in this section. Complete essays can be found in chapter 6. In an effort to be gender neutral and maintain anonymity for the writers, I've shifted between masculine and feminine pronouns when providing sample essay excerpts.

The following chart lists some potential assets to demonstrate in your essay:

Knowledge-Based Skills	Transferable Skills	Personal Skills
Intelligent	Medical Background	Energetic
Effective Problem-Solver	Military Background	Positive
Culturally Knowledgeable	Leadership Experience	Sense of Humor
Critical Thinker	Coaching Experience	Enthusiastic
Scientifically Knowledgeable	Teaching Experience	Calm
Verbally Skilled	Customer Service Rep.	Kind
Effective Presenter	Team Member	Compassionate
Second or Third Language Knowledge	Mediator	Empathic
Creative	Negotiator	Well Organized
Knowledgeable about Statistics	Worked in Underserved Areas	Effective Communicator

Review this list, think strategically about what you want to emphasize, and then step back and assess your themes.

Writing your essay will require you to put multiple themes into one short essay— which is not always easy.

There are three main themes that are necessary in admissions essays. The first theme is associated with why you want to be a PA. The second theme relates to how you are unique or exceptional. And the third main theme addresses your qualifications and experience. All three add up to: What do you bring to the profession?

Theme One: Why You Want to Be a PA

The admissions committee will want to know why you want to be a PA, because this motivation will likely influence your success and happiness in the profession. Since the PA field is not as well-known as some other health-care professions (e.g., nurse or physician), it is important that you clearly understand and then articulate your understanding of the profession in your essay.

In order to assess how to present this theme, think back on when you first realized you wanted to be a PA. How old were you? Was there a specific event that inspired you? When did you first become aware of the profession?

I've Always Wanted to Help People

Since individuals who want to be PAs generally do care for people and want to help them with their medical needs, this is a common response. While common, it can become trite and predictable, so it is important to find a creative and original way to talk about your concern for people.

The writer of essay 14 does this by talking about a career that provided less fulfill-ment than he wanted:

> My entire career had been spent working in the corporate world where all that matters is the bottom line. I needed to find a way to help others and, more impor-tantly, to make a difference.

In contrast to the previous writer, who found the PA field after being in the corpo-rate world, the writer of essay 38 has known she wanted to be a PA since she was young:

I have desired to be a physician assistant literally since the time I discovered what a PA is. Two things set in motion my dream of becoming a PA: First, I have had a desire since childhood to help people…The secondary source of inspiration came due to a meeting with and being treated by a PA at my doctor's office. Her personable and kind manner set me at ease and she was truly professional in her work.

Essay 26's writer draws on an experience with an elderly patient to emphasize both her health-care experience and her interest in helping people:

The best part of my first job was forming relationships with patients. As I prepared to draw blood from an elderly gentleman, I noticed that he had visited a doctor in another clinic that morning. When I informed him he could have had his blood drawn there instead of driving all the way across town, his response was, "I know that, but you won't screw it up." His words let me know how important it was for him to have someone he trusted draw his blood, and I felt honored to be that person. As a physician assistant, I will always be mindful that a patient's trust is an essential component of optimal healthcare.

Finally, the writer of essay 38 writes poignantly about helping people:
First I have had a desire since childhood to help people. The examples shown by both my father and grandfather as ministers were ever-present influences on the desperate need of the human heart for healing, as well as the gratification that serving them and helping in the healing process can bring. My heart was stirred to help people—I went on various missions trip with my church to a native American reservation and to Mexico and I witnessed the health needs of the people there, both physically and mentally.

A PA Changed My Life

Sometimes having a person who is in the profession impact you or someone you know becomes a reason for choosing that profession. Essays 19 and 20 detail encounters that affected their writers' interest and desire to be a PA.

From essay 19:
"A PA helped save my daughter's life" exclaimed my co-worker Christy. She detailed how the persistence and advocacy of a PA at the ER had been instrumental in diagnosing her daughter with Kawasaki syndrome. As she spoke, I was struck—yet again—by the dedication of this PA; not unlike that of the many other PAs I had contacted in prior months. Though I had been exploring the profession for some

time already, it was this defining moment that truly cemented my desire to become a PA.

From essay 20:

Two years ago, tragedy reared its ugly head again when my mother was diagnosed with saddle pulmonary embolism and was admitted at Beth Israel Hospital for two weeks. Our family was grief-stricken at the thought of losing our mother, yet nearly every visit we found her chatting good-naturedly with her PA. They developed a friendship, and I saw what a difference the PA made not only in caring for my mother's physical health but for her mental health as well. The way she accompanied my mother's every step until her recovery triggered my decision to pursue a career as a physician assistant.

Finally, the writer of essay 31 details how impressed she was by the PAs she shadowed while working as a clinician:

During my training, I learned about the physician assistant profession and, for some of my rotations, I followed a PA when the physician was not available. The broad medical knowledge, accurate diagnosis, and sharp clinical skills of one PA impressed me enormously, and I admired his dedication to his patients and his satisfaction with his career.

The Profession Is Well-Suited for Me

Another reason you might have selected the PA profession is because you saw the career as a good fit for you. In this case, you will want to identify the reasons why it is a good fit.

The writer of essay 13 also addresses this theme in the introduction and then goes on to address why the career is the right career for her. The Physician Assistant (PA) profession fulfills a unique niche in medicine:

The aspects of this career that make it so interesting and fitting for me are: the team dynamics of working with physicians, nurses, and other health care professionals, the opportunity and flexibility to work in different subspecialty areas, and the ability to spend more time with patients than the supervising physician. I particularly am drawn to the dynamic of collaborating with physicians to ensure quality care is given. The particular aspect of the PA profession I desire is the ability to be trained as a generalist and further the education to a specialty if I desire.

The writer of essay 7 addresses this issue right up front by outlining a different combination of experiences that led him to want to become a PA:

The wide-ranging experiences of nearly losing my father, volunteering, teaching middle-schoolers, and running have led to my wholehearted pursuit of a career as a physician assistant.

Theme Two: Why You Are an Exceptional Candidate

The second theme your essay needs to focus on is why you are different from the other candidates. As was previously noted, the admissions committee will have many candidates to review. You need to communicate that you are a distinctive candidate.

The writer of essay 16 uses his unique background as a tae kwon do champion to distinguish himself from other candidates:

Discovering the greatness of having a team, the joys of travel abroad, and the importance of taking care of your body, are three of the greatest gifts taekwondo has given me.

The writer of essay 24 distinguishes herself as an exceptional candidate by detailing the amount of time she has put into preparing to apply to PA school:

I have spent the last six years preparing for this application process. Having found my prefect fit, I returned to school with a focus and drive like never before.

The fact that this candidate has spent six years preparing to apply to PA school distinguishes her as a committed and serious candidate who has given the PA profession much consideration.

Essay 28 is written by someone who is currently a practicing chiropractic physician. As such, he already has a good deal of experience working with patients—a qualification that should be noted. However, an admissions committee might wonder why he would be leaving this profession. Anticipating this, he answers the question in the essay:

[Those in the chiropractic profession] seem to have so many differing philosophies and agendas that, instead of growing stronger, we have alienated ourselves from one another.

Thus, the writer distinguishes himself from other candidates with his medical background and experience yet also details what he likes about the PA profession and why he wishes to change careers.

All of these candidates find something unique to emphasize in their experiences or backgrounds that is likely to impress an admissions committee.

Theme Three: Why You Are Well Qualified

It is surprising how many people fail to emphasize their qualifications in the application essay. This is most likely because they have not completed the self-analysis I talk about in this book. Taking the time to prepare for the essay will likely alleviate an error like this.

If you do have medical experience, it is very important to emphasize that. Military experience can also be valuable as can volunteer experience, particularly if it is in the medical area.

The writer of essay 5 details his lifelong commitment to health care by elaborating on all of his health-care related experiences: high school volunteer at a local animal hospital, completion of a wilderness survival first aid and CPR course, fisheries biologist, part-time firefighter and EMT, and medical relief worker in Guatemala. While you might not think to write about your high school volunteer experiences or other opportunities you had that were many years ago, such a vast array of experiences will convince the admissions committee of your knowledge and skills.

Essays 18, 22, 26, and 27 also detail health-care experience—all from different perspectives.

The writer of essay 25, who at the time was a principal investigator for clinical trials, does an exceptional job detailing his clinical knowledge while tying his goals to the mission of the program:

> I am applying to the George Washington University Physician Assistant Program in order to advance my clinical knowledge and to gain the skills necessary to provide a higher level of patient care. Upon completion of the PA program, I plan to provide care to service-members wounded in combat and HIV/AIDS patients living in poverty, two under-served groups with which I am familiar.

All the preceding examples are written by individuals who have experiences that they can document in the essay. But what if you complete the self-analysis and find yourself without the qualifications you need? As I say in my first book: *The Ultimate*

Guide to Getting into Physician Assistant School,[8] the first step is to get some additional experience, either job-related or as a volunteer. But you can also emphasize the transferable skills we discussed earlier in this chapter.

Chapter 3 Checklist

- I have defined my goals.
- If being a PA does not seem to align with my life goals, I am reconsidering.
- I have researched the PA profession and understand the history of it.
- I have assessed various programs and considered how they might or might not be a good fit for me.
- I understand my knowledge skills.
- I understand what transferable skills I possess and know how to integrate them into my essay.
- I am aware of my personal skills.

---

8   Available at Amazon.com: http://www.amazon.com.

PART II
Writing

Ready, Set, Write

4

You have completed the preliminary steps for writing this essay. You can now begin to craft the essay, but before you do, you must consider your overall strategy.

THE FIVE CRITICAL ELEMENTS

Your goal here is to sell yourself, so you need to consider the five critical elements of your essay.

The first critical element is attention. If you don't capture your audience's attention, you can't tell them your story. And remember that your essay may be the last one they read at the end of the day, so capturing their attention is critical. I discuss attention-getting introductions in the next chapter.

Second, you need to generate interest. How are you a unique candidate? What is your story, and how is it interesting? Every human being is interesting. Even if you don't have an amazing story to tell, you can still be interesting in the way you tell your story.

Third, you need to demonstrate sincere conviction. Every other candidate will say that he or she is "passionate" about being a PA. You need to show it in a way that isn't cliché and that is sincere.

Fourth, attraction is important. You need to show that you want them badly! Attraction is a two-way street, and if you don't appear enthusiastic about them or the field, they will not be enthusiastic about you. Attraction and desire create interest, and that will further advance your cause.

Finally, you need to close the essay on a positive note. A good ending leaves the reader feeling good about the candidate and wanting to learn more about her or him. The goal of the essay is to get you an interview—so make sure that your last words of the essay ensure that it will happen.

Now that we've reviewed the five main elements of the essay, let's start writing!

OUTLINES, FREE-WRITING, MIND-MAPPING

Many people think that the best way to start an essay is to write the introduction. In truth, the introduction should be written last. So rather than sitting down and writing the introduction, it is best to start an essay with the goal of simply *getting some words on paper*. If you are still struggling, refer back to the writing warm-ups discussed previously.

Some writers can sit down and easily draft an outline of what they will write. Some writers prefer to free-write. And still another strategy involves mind-mapping. I talk about all of these in the following sections.

Outlining

You probably learned about outlining in elementary school. It is generally thought to be the preferred way to start a writing project, but it isn't for everyone. If you tend to be very organized and like step-by-step processes, you will most likely benefit from doing an outline first.

Outlining generally includes the following format:
Introduction
    I. Attention getter
    II. Overview
Body
    I. Main point I
        A. Supporting data/story I
        B. Supporting data/story 2
    II. Main point 2
        A. Supporting data/story I
        B. Supporting data/story 2
(additional points as needed)
Conclusion
    I. Summary
    II. Closing appeal
It is a good idea to start with the main points and then create the introductory information and concluding information when you have completed the body.

Free-Writing

Free-writing is wonderful for creative people or times when you have a writer's block. It helps you access a different part of the brain—which can be very helpful at starting a project or moving through a writing block.

Free-writing involves taking a clean sheet of paper, sitting down, and writing—or drawing. You can use words, phrases, or even diagrams and drawings.

It is important to *just write*. Don't critique your writing or drawing or doodling—just do it. Before you know it, you will have ideas and thoughts about your essay that you may not have known you had. When you have completed the free-writing, you can start to organize your thoughts around main ideas or topics you wish to include.

Mind-Mapping

Mind-mapping is a process by which you create a diagram to better assist you in understanding a problem or issue. For writing an admissions essay, you would map in the following manner.

First, write the title of your essay in the center of the page and draw a circle or oval around it (see figure 1). Second, begin to map the subtopics that come to mind as you think about your topic. In the case of your essay, you want to build a case for acceptance. Third, continue to dig down further until you have a complete map of your essay ideas. For instance, in this map, you might "burrow" down more on what team sports taught you about being a good team member and how this will connect with your work in the health-care profession.

Don't worry about the design of the map. The only important thing is that it makes sense to you.

Figure 1: Mind Map of Application Essay

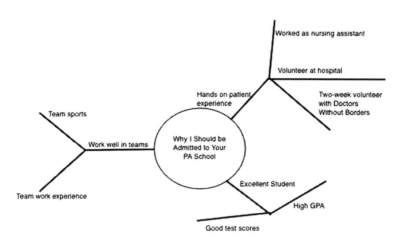

Organization

Now that you've identified what you want to talk about in the essay, it is time to organize it into a coherent piece. Do not underestimate the importance of a well-organized essay. Not only are well-organized essays easier for the reader to comprehend, they communicate to him or her that you too are organized and can communicate well—something that is critical for being an effective PA.

There are many different ways to organize your essay, but I will talk here about the three that are most applicable to the PA essay.

In a *topical* organizational pattern, you list your points or arguments without consideration to any particular order. An essay written from the mind-map example given above could be written with a topical pattern.

A variation of the topical pattern is the *more-important-to-least-important* pattern. While the essay is still topical, the writer decides which points are most and least important. Typically, the most important point comes first, the second most important point comes last, and the points of lesser importance go in the middle. The primacy/recency effect says that people tend to remember what they hear first and last, which is why you want to include those points at the beginning and end of the essay.

In a *chronological pattern* of organizing, the writer presents information in order of the timing of the events. You might include this pattern if a series of chronological events in your life led you to an interest in the PA profession.

Again, do not underestimate the power of a well-organized essay. It communicates more about your organizational skills and suitability for the rigorous training and practice of being a PA than you may be aware.

TELLING YOUR STORY: WRITING NARRATIVE

Your story. This is what will distinguish you from your competition. We are all unique and have an individual story to tell, but it is important to put the pieces of the story together for your reader. The story captures the attention of the reader and gives him or her important information about you. Consider this story from essay 1:

"Your wife is dying!" Hearing those words marked a turning point in my life. When it came time for the birth of our fourth son, financial circumstances found us without medical insurance. However, with three previously healthy deliveries, we believed a home birth with a mid-wife would be okay. The birth went great until my wife had a retained placenta. In my ignorance I calmly held my wife in my arms as she was slowly bleeding to death. When the mid-wife finally alerted us to the true nature of our situation, I hit a point of fear and desperation I had never known before. I was powerless to help my wife except to race her to the hospital where a very capable physician and staff were able to calmly administer three units of blood and confidently perform the necessary lifesaving procedures. Although life pursuits had initially taken me through other vocations, this experience became the catalyst for our family decision for me to become a Physician Assistant (PA).

In just 168 words, this essay tells a lot about the candidate's motivation for becoming a PA. It includes all the key elements of a good narrative: characters (the writer, the wife, the midwife, and the hospital staff), the setting (at home and then the hospital), the plot (having the baby at home), the conflict (the retained placenta), and the resolution (a healthy outcome).

Tips for Writing Effective Narratives

- Your narrative is only a part of the essay, so be thoughtful about length.
- Always focus on the positive. Even if the story itself isn't positive, the end should be.
- Try to use words that create images and pictures in the reader's mind. For instance, the writer in essay 1 writes: "I calmly held my wife in my arms as she was bleeding to death." A less descriptive sentence would be: "Without my realizing it, my wife was bleeding to death."
- Make certain that the narrative is important to your overall story. Don't use a story just for attention or shock value.

Remember that even if you don't have a dramatic story, you can make any story interesting and real if you develop it correctly and include all the elements of effective stories.

PARAGRAPHS AND TRANSITIONS

Paragraphs and transitions serve important functions in writing: they assist the reader in tracking the information. The last thing you want in an essay is to have the admissions committee lost when they read what you have written.

Effective paragraphs have one main point and several sentences that support that main point. The topic sentence for the paragraph usually leads but can be introduced later if you want to build suspense. The details or "proof" for the point you are trying to make follow.

As a general rule, paragraphs should be between 75 and 125 words. If you find your paragraphs getting longer, revisit to make sure you have only one main idea in the paragraph.

Transitions can consume an entire paragraph in longer writing. However, in shorter writing, like your application essay, the transition should be one sentence or even a short phrase. For instance, you can transition with "Now that I've explained to you my motivation for going to PA school, I'd like to tell you about my qualifications and background." Or you might use transitional words and phrases, such as: *additionally, in contrast, to further illustrate, in summary,* et cetera.

Read the excerpt below from essay 12, and note how clearly each paragraph is organized around one main idea. Also note the logical progression of ideas organized in chronological order.

"Rand missus?" The boy held out his tiny grimy hands, eagerly, hopefully. Most striking was the smaller child standing next to him, a gaping hole extending up from his split upper lip. I handed the boy the change I had, knowing it could do little to improve their situation, but wanting to do something. Their hopeful, expectant faces created a poignant image that remains with me, even now, 15 years later. It was during this trip to the war ravaged capital of Mozambique, as a young exchange student studying in South Africa, that I first became truly mindful of the physical consequences of poverty. I felt quite helpless at that time and wished I could do more for them. My brief encounter with them, and similar experiences while in South Africa, made me realize that I didn't want to be helpless. I wanted to make an impact in the lives of those around me. Specifically, I decided that I wanted to pursue a career path, where I could contribute to the health and well being of my community.

Returning from my studies abroad, I changed my major to Anthropology. I knew that I wanted to go into some sort of health field, and felt strongly that understanding people and the cultural context in which they exist would be a good start. I also completed all of the pre-requisites for applying to medical school. Following graduation, rather than medical school, I chose to obtain a graduate degree in public health at the University of Utah. This proved to be a natural complement to my studies in anthropology and a very rewarding experience. I really felt like I had found my niche and hoped it would provide me the opportunity to make a positive contribution to the community.

I was fortunate to get a job with the Utah Department of Health, Office of Epidemiology, in the sexually transmitted disease (STD) surveillance program.

WORD CHOICE

The most important first step in word choice is to think about the appropriate level of formality to use when you write. With the increased use of online technology, social networking, and texting, many writers fail to appreciate the importance of this consideration.

Clearly, you want a moderate to formal level of writing in an application essay. You want it personal (less formal) but professional (more formal). And you certainly don't want it to sound like a text you would send to your friends.

To ensure that your writing is appropriate, remember that informal language tends to be imprecise and can embarrass you in the hands of the wrong reader.

Consider the following guidelines for effective word choice:

- use active voice
- be specific
- avoid unnecessary jargon
- use appropriate medical terms when needed
- avoid clichés
- avoid euphemisms
- avoid "fancy" words
- make sure that you understand all terminology you use
- take care to use inoffensive language (e.g., gender neutral/nonsexist)

The writer of essay 5 uses particularly effective language in the writing. Note that the writer uses active voice, is specific, and avoids jargon and clichés.

After earning my undergraduate degree in zoology I pursued a career as a fisheries biologist, and for the past 15 years I have been involved in extended field research projects in the Bering Sea and Gulf of Alaska. Long hours, harsh conditions, and intricate scientific research challenge the best people when working on a ship. As a crew leader for the past 12 years I understand that everyone's lives depend on each other when at sea; thus, effective leadership, positive teamwork and a little humor are essential to completing the tasks while maintaining morale and retuning home safely. These life skills are applicable far beyond the ocean.

Using Writing Tools

Word processing tools present us with opportunities to avoid errors like never before. They also assist us in finding more descriptive language and avoiding unnecessary repetition in words. However, be careful when using them.

Grammar check will help you catch grammatical errors such as misplaced phrases, sentence fragments, and noun/verb conflicts.

Spellcheck works well for misspelled words, but will not correct wrong words that are spelled correctly -- e.g. "lead" versus "led," "to" versus "too," etc. So be sure to proof your writing in addition to using spellcheck.

A thesaurus can be particularly helpful when you want to avoid repetition. For instance: "I was able to assist the woman who needed assistance, even though she was already being assisted by someone else" can be changed to "I was able to lend a hand to the woman who needed assistance even though she was being helped by someone else."

Some people use the thesaurus to try to make their writing sound more sophisticated. This sentence, for instance, uses less common words: "I could tell that there was a good deal of acrimony between the PA and the nurse by the glib non sequitur response he gave him." A much clearer sentence would be: "I could tell that there was tension between the PA and the nurse by the brief and unrelated response he gave him."

In summary, a good rule of thumb is to use these tools without overusing them and without becoming completely dependent upon them for your proofing step.

INTRODUCTIONS AND CONCLUSIONS

Introductions and conclusions are critical to any writing. They tell the readers what to expect in the piece and then summarize what they have read. However, they also serve other functions. They help gain the audience's attention and also add a final call to action at the end.

Introductions should start with something that catches the readers' attention. However, it should relate to your purpose. For an application essay then, make sure that your attention getter is appropriate and relevant. You don't have the space to write something that doesn't serve to advance your cause.

Essay 10 catches the reader's attention but also explains the relevance of this otherwise unrelated story:

"Ready! Droppin' in 3...2...1," I called to the videographers and photographers below me. The whiteout conditions on that January day had hindered our filming efforts and, as the weather broke, I knew that my chances to complete the maneuver were limited. My heart raced as I looked toward the edge of the cliff, but I pushed doubt and fear from my mind and focused on making a perfect landing. With my snowboard pointing downhill, I visualized my landing and followed through with precision and confidence.

Throughout my ten-year career as a professional snowboarder, jumping off cliffs had become routine, and I believed in myself and in my abilities. Aware that hesitation results in accidents, I continually pushed myself to advance and excel. Understanding my mind and body was vital to my success, I became obsessed with health, wellness, and healing. Now, as I prepare to become a physician assistant, I approach a different cliff in my life, but the same principles of preparation, practice, commitment, and confidence still apply.

While we may not all have stories like this, we can create attention through several other strategies.

You can also start your essay with a quote. Essay 5 quotes Sir Winston Churchill: Sir Winston Churchill once said, "We make a living by what we get; we make a life by what we give."

Another strategy is to write something inspiring or write about someone who is inspiring. The writer of essay 14 uses this strategy:

Some of us are fortunate enough to have a person enter our life that has such a profound impact that it forever changes the direction of our lives. For me this was my brother-in-law's mother, Judy Hall. She had an amazing capacity for giving that was evident from the first time I met her.

Still another strategy is to create suspense. The author of essay 19 starts with: "*A PA helped save my daughter's life*" and the author of essay 2 starts with: "*Early on June 25, 2011, as Flight 3906 began its ascent, my seatmate grabbed my arm...*"

Using a personal introduction can also be effective. The writer of essay 15 uses this strategy:

At 17 my doctor diagnosed me with Scheuermann's kyphoscoliosis and a spinal curvature of 90 degrees. I underwent a full thoracic-lumbar spinal fusion...

Conclusions summarize the writing, and add a final appeal to the reader. The writer of essay 35 uses the conclusion to highlight how she/he is "uniquely suited" for the profession and to summarize her/his talents and skills:

My abilities and experiences are uniquely suited for the PA profession. I have spent my life witnessing, working, and researching medicine. This has had a profound effect upon me, not only teaching me about medicine itself, but also imbuing me with a strong sense of empathy and compassion. My curiosity, intelligence, and drive to treat the physical and emotional needs of my patients will make me an excellent PA.

The writer of essay 31 uses the conclusion to summarize her or his skills and attributes and emphasize her or his commitment to becoming a PA.

My desire and commitment to becoming a physician assistant is so strong that I will not allow any obstacles to deter my progress. I intend to make the most of every opportunity to achieve this goal, and I look forward to bringing my strong motivation, reliability, interpersonal skills, and capacity for hard work to this program.

Essay 39 gives us perhaps the best example of using an effective introduction and conclusion to create a narrative. I encourage you to look at that essay to see how an effective conclusion can leave the reader with an extremely positive closing thought and impression of the candidate.

Chapter 4 Checklist

- I used an outline, free-writing, or mind-mapping process to generate ideas for my essay.
- My essay is organized clearly—e.g., chronologically, topically, et cetera.
- If my essay is organized topically, I've put my most important points first and last.
- My stories are interesting and relevant to my application.
- Each of my paragraphs has only one main idea.

- There are clear transitions between each of my main ideas.
- I've used professional language and avoided slang and colloquialisms.
- I have an attention-getting introduction.
- I have a clear conclusion that summarizes my points and leaves the reader with a positive closing thought.

Polishing and Perfecting

5

Now that you have a good draft of your essay, it is time to step back from it a bit and consider how you will polish it to make it even stronger.

EDITING

Editing is the process of reviewing your document to be sure that all grammar, spelling, punctuation, and mechanics are correct. While word-processing programs can check for many errors, don't be led to complacency because there are some errors they won't catch. For instance, if I had written "Four instance" rather than "For instance," my spell check would not catch it. It also may not catch inaccurate name spellings and homophones like "two/too/to" and "their/there." In other words, don't trust it alone.

Common errors to watch for include: sentence fragments, comma splices, run-on sentences, ambiguous pronouns, unclear comparisons, subject-verb agreement mismatches, inaccurate tense use, passive voice use, and incorrect colon versus semicolon use.

Here are some examples of these typical errors:

* *This was a difficult time for the patient. Especially difficult due to his advanced disease.* (The second phrase is a sentence fragment)
* *This was a difficult time for the patient, he was very ill.* (comma splice)
* *This was a difficult time for the patient who was ill and he was not able to communicate his needs to the nurses and doctors.* (run-on sentence)
* *The patient was very ill and told the doctor about the symptoms. He was not very clear.* (ambiguous pronoun).
* This was a difficult time for the patient. He is very ill. (inaccurate tense use).
* *The patient was very ill. Were he to explain this to the doctor, his condition would have improved.* (passive voice use)
* *This was a difficult time for the patient; he was very ill.* (colon/semi-colon misuse)

If in doubt, buy a good grammar book or look up common grammar problems online for helpful tips. You can also hire someone to edit and proofread your essay.

PROOFREADING

Proofreading is the process of checking your document to make sure you have typed what you meant to type. The common errors for spell check mentioned above are what to look for when proofreading.

Also, realize that our perceptions influence how we proofread. For instance, read this sentence quickly:

The flowers in Paris are

are lovely in the Springtime.

If you read it quickly, you may have missed the fact that there is more than one "are." Our perceptions influence how we see our writing when we proofread. Some writing experts suggest that we proofread backward to avoid being lulled into complacency by our perceptions and expectations.

REVISIONS

Editing and proofing are parts of creating revisions, but revisions also include looking at the essay from the larger perspective.

Revisions can be difficult because it is sometimes hard to take a fresh look at your writing and spot problems. But there are three main things to examine.

The first is related to audience. Sometimes the process of writing provides you with an opportunity to think more clearly about your audience. Ask yourself if writing the essay has caused you to change your ideas about your readers. If so, what do you need to change now that you have a different understanding of the people who will read your work?

Second, is your purpose still the same? You may have started writing your essay with the intention of getting into PA school based upon your good grades, but maybe after writing it, you discovered other strengths that you should emphasize instead. If so, reexamine the essay to make sure that all of the parts clearly work toward your newly defined purpose, and if you discover they do not, revise.

Finally, has your perception of your subject changed? Since you are the subject for this essay, the process of writing may have provided you with new ideas about yourself.

If so, make sure that they are integrated into the essay and that you are communicating a consistent message about the subject—you.

HONESTY AND ACCURACY

Getting admitted to PA school is a competitive endeavor. Consequently, it is sometimes tempting to overstate your qualifications—to "fudge" a bit on the details of your background. *Don't do it!*

Not only is it not right, it will backfire on you. The purpose of the essay is to get you to the interview at a school. If you lie or mislead on the essay, it *will* come out in the interview.

So, do a fact check to make sure that what you say is accurate. Did you really learn all that you said you did from that experience working with a certain group of patients? Was your GPA as high as you claim it was? Are you really as knowledgeable as you say you are about certain patient care? While it is not necessary (or effective) to understate your abilities/skills/knowledge, overstatement will get you into trouble later.

TONE

This is also a good time to check for tone. Do you come across as sufficiently humble? The committee will want to know that you are willing to learn. Sounding overly confident in the essay will be a red flag for the committee.

On the other hand, being too tentative will not help create a good impression either. Some writers (especially women) use the phrases "I think" or "I believe" repeatedly, for example: "*I think* I am well suited for the PA profession because..." Rather than being tentative about the statement, it is better to say: "I am well suited for the PA profession because..."

CLARITY

Clear writing ensures that the review committee understands your message easily. They have a good idea of who you are, why you are interested in being a PA, and why you would be a good addition to their program.

To be sure your message is clear, reread your essay aloud. Does it make sense? Have you "filled in all the blanks"? If you were on an admissions committee, what remaining questions would you have?

The writer of essay 2 has a very powerful story to tell but omits an important element and leaves the reader a bit confused. We are able to fill in the gaps eventually, but catching omissions like this can be very important to the writing process:

I told the flight attendant that Garrett needed emergency medical attention, and an RN came forward to help. I reported my findings to the nurse, who assumed control of communication with the flight crew. When Garrett was no longer able to sit upright, we lay him on the cabin floor and swabbed his face with wet towels, but his pain was relentless. His lips were white and his pupils dilated; at times he became verbally unresponsive. When we finally reached the Charlotte airport, no ambulance or emergency team awaited us. After we landed, the RN walked away from the patient, and first responders rebuffed my efforts to communicate with them, so I also walked away and hurried to catch my next flight. That night, Garrett died.

Months later, I sat in a stuffy conference room, responding to questions from a USAirways investigator. After two hours of questioning, her tone changed, her voice hardened, and she asked suspiciously, "Why did you call his parents?" I stared at the red light on the tape recorder and tried to compose my thoughts. It occurred to me that she thought I might be looking for compensation. "My brother was killed when he was 18," I said. "I've seen what happens to parents when their children die. They have questions. Most of all, they ask, 'When my child was suffering, did anyone help him? When he was in pain, was there someone with him who cared?'"

It would have been helpful to the reader if the writer mentioned that after she heard of the young man's death, she made a point to call his parents to tell them what she had seen. Reading your own work as if it is the first time you've read it can be helpful in catching gaps in stories.

If the message isn't completely clear or has gaps, rewrite.

CONCISENESS

Now comes the hard part. You have slaved over every word and thought in the essay, and it is too long. Now is the time you must cut and edit.

Disciplined cutting is essential to an effective essay. Cutting can make you feel like you are wasting the time you spent writing the words in the first place and thus may be hard. This is important: *Good writers are merciless with cutting their pieces.*

Here is an excerpt from essay 28 before and after cutting:

Before:

I am currently looking to make a change in my career. The last few years have been a time for me to reflect, review my career objectives, and plan for change, with a focus on reviewing my career objectives. I have come to the conclusion that I want to be involved in a career with a promising that has a bright future and, is directly involved with people. My future career must be in the medical arena, meet my need for continuing education, provide me with an opportunity for change, and will use my past life experiences, training, and work experiences and skills. The physician associate profession meets that all of those criteria. There is no question as to the viability of the physician assistant profession. Certainly, the creation of a national health care system that that demands affordable health care will only increase the need for PA's, and the need. Indicators predict that the PA profession will be around for the next decade and beyond. I still have another 20 to 25 twenty to twenty-five working years of work ahead of me, and I want my next profession to be one that will offer both challenge and a lot of opportunity.

After:

The last few years have been a time for me to reflect, review my career objectives, and plan for change. I want a medical career with a promising future and direct involvement with people. My future career must meet my need for continuing education, provide an opportunity for change, and utilize my past life experiences, training, and skills. The physician associate profession meets that criteria, and the viability of the physician assistant profession is without question. The creation of a national healthcare system that demands affordable healthcare will only intensify the need for PA's, and indicators suggest that this profession will grow throughout the next decade and beyond. I still have twenty to twenty-five working years ahead of me, and I want my next profession to be one that will offer both challenge and opportunity.

Not only is the revision more succinct and clear, this writer cut out nearly seventy words between version one and two thus allowing for more space to write about other attributes the applicant would bring to the profession.

Chapter 5 Checklist

- My essay is free of grammatical, spelling, usage, and other errors.
- My essay is free of typographical mistakes.

- The information in my essay is honest and communicates an accurate picture of who I am and my skills.
- The tone of my essay is appropriate for an admissions committee audience.
- Each of my paragraphs has only one main idea.
- My writing is clear and understandable.
- My writing is succinct.
- I have been merciless in my edits and cuts.

6

Sample Essays

In this chapter, you will find sample essays from others who have gone through this process. All of the writers of these essays were asked to interview for at least one school of their choice.

These essays are meant to assist you by giving you examples from which to learn. You may like aspects of some essays and not like aspects of others. Some have errors—grammatical and otherwise—so see if you can catch those and then recognize how easy it is to submit an essay with errors.

Plagiarizing from these essays is illegal. As I said, they are provided for you as tools which you can use to learn to write a quality essay.

Essay 1 (826 words)

"Your wife is dying!" Hearing those words marked a turning point in my life. When it came time for the birth of our fourth son, financial circumstances found us without medical insurance. However, with three previously healthy deliveries, we believed a home birth with a mid-wife would be okay. The birth went great until my wife had a retained placenta. In my ignorance I calmly held my wife in my arms as she was slowly bleeding to death. When the mid-wife finally alerted us to the true nature of our situation, I hit a point of fear and desperation I had never known before. I was powerless to help my wife except to race her to the hospital where a very capable physician and staff were able to calmly administer three units of blood and confidently perform the necessary lifesaving procedures. Although life pursuits had initially taken me through other vocations, this experience became the catalyst for our family decision for me to become a Physician Assistant (PA).

Entering the world of the PA is an incredible challenge. I have overcome other incredible challenges before, especially when I walked onto the men's gymnastic team as a freshman in college. Because my last gymnastics class was in elementary school, I lacked the basic training and experience of my teammates. Yet, what I lacked in preparation I made up for with passion and dedication. I did not compete as a gymnast my first year on the team but I was determined to succeed. The following years I did compete as a part of our championship team and was the team captain my senior year. Like my experience with the gymnastic team, I am confident that I can handle the rig-ors, work ethic, and commitment required to become a champion PA.

Being a part of the community and helping others thrive has always been a driv-ing force in my life. Growing up on the Navajo Indian Reservation there were ample opportunities to serve. Organizing church and Boy Scout service projects designed to improve our community were regular activities for me. Formally and informally, I tutored friends and peers in high school and college. Later, as a real estate agent, I found great joy and satisfaction in helping families find their way to owning their first homes. As I did in the Upward Bound programs of my high school, I have always worked to help members of my community improve their circumstances and strive for better things in life.

Being a PA is the best way to focus my desire to improve and help my community in a meaningful way with my passion for excellence. When I was growing up on the Reservation, there was only a two-room clinic with a rotating doctor and reception-ist. Frequently, we traveled hours just to get into a town with a fully staffed clinic and modern healthcare facilities and equipment. Being a PA would make it possible to take full-time help back to the reservation and to other towns in similar situations. So many of my friends deal with chronic pains and problems that may have been prevented with current medical care. As a PA, I will have the training to help care for my friends, fam-ily, and community, and to break the poor health cycle by helping their children have a better quality of life.

Once my family and I realized that becoming a PA was the route I should take, we took immediate action. I quit my job and returned to school full-time to take the PA program pre-requisite coursework as quickly as possible. I also took the time to acquire patient care experience. My patient care experience has been an opportunity to work with mentally ill patients—a significant population of medically underserved people right here in our communities. Because of my driving desire to help, I have frequently been with my patients six and seven days a week often volunteering to stay late, picking up extra shifts, and working on all of the units in the hospital. It has been satisfying and fulfilling for me to see so many of my patients go from their deepest problems to developing a significant measure of mental health and control and being discharged from the hospital to return to society.

The exciting and challenging world of a healthcare provider and the rewarding career as a Physician Assistant is about being able to care for people, especially the underserved members of our community. I want to spend my life caring for people who really need and deserve quality healthcare. Once trained, I will be able to take my medical experience back to the Reservation, and to other deserving communities as well. While my life has taken some interesting turns, I am someone who is prepared for the academic rigors, the strict work ethic, the compassion for patients, and the caring to reach out to our community that makes for a truly great PA.

Essay 2 (940 words)

Early on June 25, 2011, as Flight 3906 began its ascent, my seatmate grabbed my arm. "There's something wrong with that boy," she warned. "I think he may be having an anxiety attack." In the seat behind me, Garrett, sweat running down his face, leaned forward and clutched his abdomen. Calling on my training as an EMT and a technician in Yale-New Haven Hospital's Emergency Department, and remembering countless conversations with my husband, an ED physician, I did a quick assessment and gathered a history. This 16-year-old was very sick, and when the plane reached altitude minutes later, Garrett's pulse became rapid and irregular.

I told the flight attendant that Garrett needed emergency medical attention, and an RN came forward to help. I reported my findings to the nurse, who assumed control of communication with the flight crew. When Garrett was no longer able to sit upright, we lay him on the cabin floor and swabbed his face with wet towels, but his pain was relentless. His lips were white and his pupils dilated; at times he became verbally unresponsive. When we finally reached the Charlotte airport, no ambulance or emergency team awaited us.

After we landed, the RN walked away from the patient, and first responders rebuffed my efforts to communicate with them, so I also walked away and hurried to catch my next flight. That night, Garrett died.

Months later, I sat in a stuffy conference room, responding to questions from a USAirways investigator. After two hours of questioning, her tone changed, her voice hardened, and she asked suspiciously, "Why did you call his parents?" I stared at the red light on the tape recorder and tried to compose my thoughts. It occurred to me that she thought I might be looking for compensation. "My brother was killed when he was 18," I said. "I've seen what happens to parents when their children die. They have questions. Most of all, they ask, 'When my child was suffering, did anyone help him? When he was in pain, was there someone with him who cared?'"

Had I been in that situation a few years earlier, I would have wanted to help, but with no training, I would have held back. I probably would not have realized how sick he really was.

Just a few years before that flight, I had been a public relations executive, helping to grow a business from $6 million to $70 million in five years. I worked hard and was good at my job, but I felt no passion for it. For emotional fulfillment, I looked outside my job. I volunteered on political campaigns, assisted with communication efforts to fight my neighborhood's epidemic of teen suicide, and tutored inner-city students. All of this ended in catastrophe. In 2006, my company restructured, and I lost my high-paying job. My house flooded. I became very ill, and my oncologist performed surgery. Two days later, I hemorrhaged and received last rites and additional emergency surgery. My father, who was brilliant, funny, and the rock of my life, died.

Stripped of all pretense, income, and power, I was completely humbled, but it was oddly liberating. Suddenly, I was free to question the trajectory of my life, and I wondered how I had strayed so far from my ideals. I didn't know how I could find my way back. By coincidence, I heard of an EMT training program at Northeastern University. I enrolled, passed the entrance exam, applied to and entered nursing school. I fought hard for a job as an ED Tech at Yale-New Haven Hospital, and I secured that position. At YNHH, I discovered many things about myself and realized I had a talent for spotting the very sick. Having suffered the indignities of failure, poor judgment, illness, and powerlessness, I had developed genuine compassion for the poor and the disenfranchised. I sat for hours with mentally ill, alcoholic, and addicted patients. I held their hands and sometimes endured their angry insults. I bandaged wounds and dried tears. I cleaned up blood and excrement. I made mistakes and learned from them. To paraphrase Martin Luther King, I felt the arc of my own moral universe bending slowly toward justice.

At Yale-New Haven Hospital, I was part of a team of dedicated and exceptionally capable people, from physicians to nurses, technicians, and physician assistants. I became intrigued by the work of PAs and the integration of the physician's practice with that of the PA. I learned about the differential diagnosis model and its contrast with the nursing diagnosis paradigm that I continued to find so alien. I believed my choices were limited because I had made mistakes in college and had not wanted to endure the sacrifice of medical school and residency. Although I was already in nursing school when I worked at YNHH, I began to formulate plans for becoming a PA. When my husband and I moved to Kentucky, I enrolled in pre-requisite classes for PA programs.

Some have questioned why I would take on the burdens of a PA career at an age when others are seeking freedom and leisure. In response, I think of the words of author David Foster Wallace: "Of course there are all different kinds of freedom," he said, "and the kind that is most precious you will not hear much talked about in the great outside world of winning, achieving, and displaying. The really important kind of freedom involves attention, awareness, discipline, and effort, and being truly able to care about other people and to sacrifice for them, over and over, in myriad, petty, unsexy ways, every day. That is real freedom."

Essay 3 (671 words)

The dictionary defines cancer as a malignant growth that spreads destructively, yet after my diagnosis with thyroid cancer in 2008 and subsequent treatment and recuperation, I made a positive discovery. It was through my experience with radia-tion therapy that I first encountered the physician assistant profession. Growing up in rural Wyoming, my only exposure to healthcare was the traditional physician-and-nurse model. My experience as a cancer patient was the first time a practitioner other than a physician was partially responsible for my treatment. My consultation with the PA was very thorough; he took the time to get to know me on a personal level and developed a connection with me prior to my meeting with the doctor. While highly educated and professional, the physician did not have the same rapport with me that the PA had developed. The PA took the time to make me feel comfortable with him, helped me understand my scheduled treatment, and explained the process of healing following my treatment.

I am fascinated by the functions of the healthy human body as well as its healing capacity when recovering from injury, disease, neglect, or abuse; the human body and spirit are truly miraculous healers. I have been interested in science and medicine since high school when my mother was attending nursing school and having me quiz her in preparation for her upcoming exams. From that point on, I knew I wanted a career in medicine. Enrolled in college, I followed a pre-professional track that culminated with a degree in Kinesiology and Health Promotion.

After graduating from the University of Wyoming, I traveled, gained new experi-ences, and found a job working in occupational health. Although I enjoyed it, I worked alone and traveled to a new site every couple of days. This was a lonely experience and did not provide the opportunity to build new relationships or foster old ones, so I changed jobs and took a position as a personal fitness instructor. I had a variety of clients, each with their own needs and expectations; some were rehabilitating from an injury, some were working to prevent injury, and others wanted to improve their health and fitness. I learned a great deal and enjoyed working one-on-one with individuals to address their problems and help improve their lives. Although this was an enjoyable experience, I felt it was still not the right fit for me.

In 2008, I took the opportunity to work at a pediatric dental office. During my time there, I was fortunate to work directly with patients on a daily basis. This afforded me the opportunity to get to know the patients as more than simply "the crown in room 2" or "the cleaning in room 5," as I had heard the staff refer to them. I became acquainted with them on a personal level, developed a rapport, and helped them through their procedures. One patient in particular was terrified of getting an injec-tion, and I was able to keep her calm and comfort her during the procedure; now she is no longer terrified of the dentist and requests my presence at her visits. Empathizing with a patient during a difficult time means a great deal to me as a healthcare provider, and this motivates me to pursue a career as a PA.

The most important issues for patients are to feel they have been heard and to know their concerns have been addressed; four years of patient and client interaction have enabled me to become an excellent listener. Using this skill, I have found that patients will provide necessary information while developing a positive relationship with their healthcare provider. Having a flexible career in the healthcare field with multiple opportunities for service is what motivates me establish a career as a PA. My goal is to work in a rural location where I can build a practice, raise my family, and become an active member of my community. I am confident I will be an excellent PA and will always be grateful for this opportunity.

Essay 4 (751 words)

180 degrees:

The Academy Awards for advertising was a black-tie gala event held in Washington, D.C. I held three gold "Addys" in my right hand and two silver ones in my left, yet I had never felt so unfulfilled in my life. As I recalled the goal I had set twenty-three years earlier, to pursue a medical career, I saw that event as my personal tipping point.

0 degrees:

As an Airman at the David Grant Medical Center, the combination of working closely with administrators and medical staff while attending to patients provided me with an excellent introduction to healthcare. Observing the dynamics of hospital administration allowed me to experience the politics, ethics, and multidisciplinary team functions of the medical and support staff. In an organization that discourages fraternization between officers and enlisted personnel, the work of physician assistants (PA) resonated with me. The PAs seemed to connect with both groups while earning the respect and admiration of staff and patients, and this is something I had personally experienced from the perspective of a patient. As an anxious eighteen-year-old inpatient, a PA treated my injury and reassured me I would not be disciplined for the situation that had caused it. I never forgot how he took the time to listen, empathize, and make me laugh about my circumstances.

90 degrees:

While working at Danbury Hospital after leaving the Air Force, I focused on a degree in Hospital Administration, but a mentor convinced me to pursue a career in marketing. As a Grey Advertising account executive (AE), I expanded my leadership and soft skills. As the liaison between agency and client, I managed multiple projects from inception to completion in stressful, high-pressure, time-sensitive situations. I also became adept at translating and presenting an idea or strategy to clients, and I found myself naturally comfortable when working with senior executives and diverse teammates. I enjoyed leading and participating in teams and working with interesting individuals who possessed a broad assortment of skills while, together, we produced great products for our clients and achieved agency goals.

270 degrees:

After thirteen years in advertising, I yearned for a career that would allow me to become deeply involved with individual wellness and healthcare. Changing my career will only make sense if my past work experiences and skills can be utilized in the transition. Every AE knows that, to become successful, one must be multifaceted and able to anticipate the needs of the client. This philosophy parallels a PA's role as a healthcare provider and has prepared me for the PA profession. My return to medicine began with sacrificing a steady salary, attending college, working as an EMT, and volunteering as a physical therapist's aide, a nurse's aide, and a patient advocate/medical assistant at Shepherd's Clinic. Maintaining many regular PA follows, subscribing to PA journals, joining PA organizations, and continuing to read numerous PA-related books, such as A *Kernel in the Pod,* has reinforced my determination to join this profession.

I have always enjoyed giving back to my community, but volunteering at Shepherd's Clinic changed my life. Working with PAs and patients in a near-universal healthcare environment has been rewarding and fulfilling, and it has inspired me to use my education and work experience to provide the highest quality of healthcare. In the Air Force, no one has to pay for medical treatment, and the clinic provides free clinical and wellness care for indigenous and underserved patients. During my first PA follow, I met a gentleman named Jimmy during his first visit to the clinic. Jimmy had been released from prison after serving thirteen years and required a battery of tests and treatments. He now calls regularly and specifically asks for me, hoping to learn more about the clinic's latest wellness programs or just have a quick chat. Jimmy has kept his promises to maintain his therapy, find employment, and live his life as an integral part of the community.

360 degrees:

Someone told me that my life has now come full circle. Just as Jimmy resumed his life with a new passion for well-being, my passion, as a PA, is to help others achieve good health and wellness. As a PA student, I will challenge myself to produce the equivalent of five Addys for each patient and for the PA profession. Adding PA skills to my leadership and administrative experience will provide an excellent foundation for the achievement of my long-term goal of creating and practicing in primary care facilities similar to the Shepherd's Clinic.

Essay 5 (754 words)

Sir Winston Churchill once said, "We make a living by what we get; we make a life by what we give." Without knowing it, the sentiment of this quote has guided me throughout my adult life towards what I feel is my destiny: to become a physician assistant.

I first felt this inner drive as a high school teenager with an interest in veterinary medicine, which prompted me to volunteer at local animal hospitals. There I developed the skill of providing thoughtful medical attention to patients who could not convey their symptoms with words. The level of empathy, compassion, and patience required to work with animals has stayed with me, and it is at the core of my patient care skills today. This same energy made itself known once again as a young adult in college; when many of my peers were involved in social activism, I joined them but decided that I could be of best service as a street medic. I quickly developed skills in treating people using the limited means I had available. The level of focus, drive, and quick-thinking necessary to assist the injured inspired and motivated me. I wanted more.

At the completion of a course in wilderness survival first aid, I was offered the opportunity to teach the course. My instructor always told me that teaching is learning twice, which I took to heart. I became a certified instructor and not only taught the course to mountaineers but also taught CPR to various organizations and school groups, taught marine safety survival to coworkers and fellow mariners, and developed a Spanish CPR curriculum for the Latino community in my district. I continue teaching today, having developed a strong passion for sharing medical and survival information.

After earning my undergraduate degree in zoology I pursued a career as a fisheries biologist, and for the past 15 years I have been involved in extended field research projects in the Bering Sea and Gulf of Alaska. Long hours, harsh conditions, and intricate scientific research challenge the best people when working on a ship. As a crew leader for the past 12 years I understand that everyone's lives depend on each other when at sea; thus, effective leadership, positive teamwork and a little humor are essential to completing the tasks while maintaining morale and retuning home safely. These life skills are applicable far beyond the ocean.

Seven years ago I felt yet another pull to be of service and became a part-time fire fighter EMT. In this role, I find that patient care continues to be the most intriguing aspect of the job. We are given the trust to enter people's homes, to have their personal lives revealed and to effectively make quick medical assessments while providing comfort and reassurance. The only frustration in the pre-hospital emergency setting is the limited diagnostic tools and treatment options available to us, and often I find myself wishing we could do more for our patients. Our patient contact ends when we transfer care to the emergency room staff, leaving me curious as to the outcome of our initial treatment and what, if anything, we could have done to help more.

In 2010, I participated in a medical relief project in Guatemala. As a Latina born in Chile and fluent in Spanish, my initial tasks were to assist in translation between the patients and doctors. However, as the clinic became more hectic it was clear that I could and should do more. I used my EMT skills to quickly triage the patients and perform more in-depth initial assessments ahead of the doctors, which increased our efficiency. The day the lead physician asked me, "Have you ever considered a career as a PA?" was the day that changed my life. I began to learn everything about the profession, and having now thoroughly explored the physician assistant career and having gained valuable knowledge from my various PA job shadows, it is clear to me that this is the career I want for the rest of my life.

I am eager to bring the skills I have gathered from all aspects of my life to the PA profession and I look forward to being part of a medical team in a collaborative environment between doctors, nurses, and other PAs contributing to the ultimate goal of effective health care for our patients. I eagerly await the challenges and rewards of this career and know that I will gain tremendous personal satisfaction from having given the best care possible to my patients.

Essay 6 (393 words)

Several years ago, I had the opportunity to reevaluate my life plans. I realized I wanted to begin a career in the medical field, and entered a medical assisting program. During the training, I learned of various medical careers, and became captivated with the physician assistant profession. I discovered it is one of the few medical professions that not only allows involvement in patient care, but also in diagnosis and treatment.

At present, I work in a family practice office as a back office medical assistant and scribe. This means that I also have the opportunity to work alongside the doctor during each office visit. I add history, diagnoses, physical exam details and treatment plans to the office visit note while the doctor is performing the exam. Meanwhile, I also scan the electronic medical record for information that would be important to that particular visit. For example, when the doctor is considering certain medications that may affect kidney function, I look to ensure the patient has no diminished kidney function on recent lab results. I question the patient and doctor for clarification, and I propose diagnostic tests or treatments for the doctor's consideration. Observing the doctor's ability to determine when a firm hand or compassionate hand is needed has also been extremely enlightening.

I have also had the occasion to see the healthcare field from a patient's perspective. A recent diagnosis of simultaneous ovarian cancer and endometrial cancer has allowed me to see the difference a compassionate caregiver can make to a patient who is in the midst of a serious diagnosis. It has also taught me the value of early diagnosis and treatment.

I currently live in a medically underserved rural area, and understand many of the challenges of such an area. In particular, I am reminded of one elderly diabetic patient who could not afford to drive the few miles to pick up his insulin at the office where I worked. I brought it to his tiny house on my way home. That day, he also asked me for information on diabetic diets; I brought a book to him the next day.

I would prefer to work in family practice as a physician assistant where I could care for patients with varied conditions and backgrounds. I look forward to future challenges and rewards of a lifelong career as a physician assistant.

Essay 7 (500 words)

The wide-ranging experiences of nearly losing my father, volunteering, teaching middle-schoolers and running have led to my wholehearted pursuit of a career as a physician assistant.

The most powerful experience of my life was when my father was mistreated for Lyme disease, suffered a subdural hematoma, and underwent emergency brain surgery. We were told that his odds were long, but I thank God and the medical team for his full recovery. Above any other, this experience called me to action and motivated me to pursue a career as a physician assistant where I hope to provide the kind of quality care that my dad received.

My interest in healthcare and helping others was brewing long before my father's illness, however, and I was raised to work hard in pursuit of my passions. In middle school and high school, I volunteered at a hospital and nursing home where I relished my interactions with patients as I provided basic care observed the skilled physician assistants. Though I obviously lacked the technical skills to provide more direct patient care, I learned to build relationships with patients and work alongside medical staff. In college, I directly cared for patients as a personal care attendant and I was hooked; I wanted to utilize my skills to the greatest impact.

Given my passion for new experiences, after college I chose a challenging new path. Armed with only confidence, I took a two-year position as a middle school teacher in a low-income school where I taught teenagers about their bodies, encouraged budding scientists, and led my students and the science department to success. Surprisingly, it was through this experience that I discovered a new angle on my passion for medicine; witnessing the lack of healthcare available to these low-income families was my calling to effect change in the medical field. This two-year teaching commitment gave me a deep understanding of the obstacles of the underprivileged and taught me how to educate a reluctant audience while persevering against challenges.

My classroom work was largely external, but in an internal way, my passion for running has impacted my outlook and my attitude on personal health and preventative care. Through college track and running everything from 5k's to marathons, I'm fascinated by the human body. My pursuit of running and wellness has led me to work with friends and family on their personal fitness goals, which has fed my inquisitiveness about the body while improving my ability to educate others on preventative health and wellness. While internal motivation is critical, to gain more direct clinical experience I am now an emergency room volunteer where I observe staff making make decisions under extreme stress. This exposure only furthered my desire to pursue a career as a physician assistant.

My journey to pursuing my physician assistant degree has involved events and experiences that have given me tremendous appreciation for the role that PA's play in the healthcare continuum. I look forward to taking the next step in this journey to serve others.

Essay 8 (774 words)

"A 73-year-old Caucasian male is brought to the Emergency Room. He appears weak and lethargic. His family members state that they found him in this condition in his apartment and that he has likely not been eating or drinking much over the past two days. What are the patient's principal problems? How would you proceed to treat this patient?"

This is the clinical case that was presented to us during the first day of the Human Pathophysiology and Translational Science (HPTM) PhD program at the University of Texas Medical Branch (UTMB) in September 2011. The graduate program trains scientists to communicate effectively with clinicians and to accelerate the application of basic science discovery from "bench to bedside". This program gave me a special opportunity to join medical students in their courses and clinical encounters for the first six months, focusing primarily on scientific laboratory-based research.

My interest in becoming a physician assistant began in 2010 when I saw a PA for a skin infection. Because of my curiosity about his role, he invited me to observe him for several days; I was impressed by the time he took with patients and the outstanding care he provided, and I was instantly drawn to patient care. As I was completing my master's degree in biomedical science, I gained more direct experience with patients by shadowing more PAs and volunteering in hospitals and community centers. I applied to several PA programs that same year, but unfortunately did not receive an acceptance offer. I was crestfallen and unsure whether to re-apply immediately to PA schools or to continue with a PhD program. Ultimately, I enrolled in UTMB's HPTM PhD program because of the inclusion of clinical work in its curriculum.

Our first courses were gross anatomy and radiology, and by the second week we had dissected the thorax, including the anterior chest wall and breast, pleural cavity and lungs, heart and great vessels. The complexity of the human body fascinated me and I was absolutely hooked. We learned how to identify pathology found on human cadavers, learned to read X-rays and computed tomography scans, bone scans and magnetic resonance imaging to better understand the pathophysiology of diseases. In Problem-Based Learning (PBL) classes, being part of a team that analyzed clinical cases to properly diagnose patients improved my critical thinking skills and taught me how to formulate relevant questions. The intensity and fast pace of the classes was sometimes overwhelming, but strong study skills helped me succeed and enjoy six months of medical school. Moreover, I have had the privilege to observe and scrub in for surgical procedures including mastectomy and removal of liposarcoma. In addition to the PBL classes, the opportunity to join Dr. Chao in her weekly oncological conferences and to listen to doctors across various specialties discuss complicated cases deepened my knowledge and sharpened my problem solving skills.

Though I gained a great deal from this experience, what I enjoyed most was working in a collaborative and high-energy environment, as well as having direct contact with patients—opportunities that simply do not exist inside a scientific laboratory. Thus, I withdrew from the PhD program to pursue a career about which I am truly passionate: becoming a physician assistant. I immediately began shadowing more PAs, I joined the American Academy of Physician Assistants and the Texas Academy of Physician Assistants, and volunteered with the Ronald McDonald House to care for critically ill children. Observing Mr. Celis, a surgical PA at Shriners Burns Hospital, also helped me better understand the aspects of the profession. I was impressed by his autonomy in seeing patients for pre- and post-operative care and in performing minor surgeries. I have also witnessed great PA-physician teamwork through watching a coronary artery bypass surgery operated by Mr. Bratovich, a cardiothoracic surgical PA, with the attending surgeon at the Methodist Hospital in Houston Medical Center. In addition to my clinical exposure to the work of PA's, reading the Journal of the American Academy of Physician Assistants keeps me current about the profession's news and topics. Additionally, I am taking a physiology course and will soon be enrolling in a medical Spanish class.

These experiences have only deepened my desire to pursue a physician assistant career. Since I first applied to PA programs I am more mature, focused, determined and motivated to succeed in an intense curriculum. I wish to integrate and utilize my scientific training and medical background to excel as a student and to become an outstanding healthcare provider. Trained in your rigorous program, I look forward to ultimately becoming a compassionate physician assistant who makes a true difference in the lives of my patients.

Essay 9 (706 words)

My first encounter with a PA occurred during an EMT course as a senior in high school. The clinical rotation required for the course provided me with a fascinating look into a world I wanted to be a part of. I remember being not only impressed, but also inspired by the story of a PA named Jim. He had been a Navy Corpsman assigned to a Marine unit in Vietnam. He explained how his military training and experience had translated into a rewarding career in the civilian world as a PA and what a great fit it was for his personality and medical groundwork. When he described his scope of practice and skill set, I knew then and there that was going to be my goal. I would use Jim's example as a template for my own career. My vocational path is not identical to Jim's, but my entire adult life has been dedicated to working in healthcare.

The first step for me was enlisting in the Air Force upon graduation from high school. Early in my career, I was trained as an Independent Duty Medical Technician (IDMT). Although the scope of practice of an IDMT and a PA are vastly different, there is one important similarity—IDMTs are trained to work autonomously in austere conditions under the guidance of a physician. This methodology simultaneously promotes independent practice and a team concept.

As an example of this concept in action, I was deployed as the senior medic for a 90-person construction project in the island nation of St. Kitts. The junior Navy Corpsman deployed with me asked for a consult on a patient who had been experiencing knee pain for 3 days, unrelieved by non-steroidal, anti-inflammatory medications (NSAIDS). Upon examination, I noted that the calf of the affected leg was larger than that of the non-affected leg. After a thorough exam and comprehensive history, I consulted my physician preceptor with concerns of a deep vein thrombosis (DVT) and requested authorization for an ultrasound, which was approved and subsequently revealed a very large clot in the popliteal vein. Even though the likelihood of a DVT was slim, my instinct, training, and experience resulted in prompt treatment and averted a potentially life-threatening complication.

During my 20-year military career, I was deployed numerous times, from the first Gulf War to Operation Iraqi Freedom. I was always proud of my service because I knew I made a difference and without me some of those men and women might not have come home. I chose to retire after 20 years and 7 months of service when the realization that my next promotion, which was inevitable, would mean I was no longer going to be involved in patient care, and I would be relegated to a strictly administrative function.

My military experience has provided me with the maturity and life experiences that will allow me to adapt well to the rigorous scholastic environment of the Physician Assistant program. In the beginning, I hit a few bumps grade wise because the shift from "real life" to the academic world proved to be a challenging transition. After joining several study groups, my study skills and confidence improved dramatically over the next few months. My extensive experience in a clinical setting will also be a huge benefit during clinical rotations. A lesson learned early in my career was that in order to be a good leader, you must first be a good follower. I earned numerous awards and decorations during my time in the Air Force, including two Meritorious Service Awards, a Humanitarian Service Award, and several Airman, Noncommissioned Officer, and Senior Noncommissioned Officer of the Quarter Awards.

Although any career in healthcare is rewarding, I hope to fulfill my lifelong goal of becoming a PA and reaching the lofty heights achieved by my inspiration Jim. Upon graduation from PA school, it is my intention to apply for a job with either the Veterans Administration or with a military facility as a contracted provider. I know I have more to give back to the military and feel the best way to do that is to continue to provide the best healthcare possible to the men and women of the Armed Services and our Veterans.

Essay 10 (825 words)

"Ready! Droppin' in 3...2...1," I called to the videographers and photographers below me. The whiteout conditions on that January day had hindered our filming efforts and, as the weather broke, I knew that my chances to complete the maneuver were limited. My heart raced as I looked toward the edge of the cliff, but I pushed doubt and fear from my mind and focused on making a perfect landing. With my snowboard pointing downhill, I visualized my landing and followed through with precision and confidence.

Throughout my ten-year career as a professional snowboarder, jumping off cliffs had become routine, and I believed in myself and in my abilities. Aware that hesitation results in accidents, I continually pushed myself to advance and excel. Understanding my mind and body was vital to my success, and I became obsessed with health, wellness, and healing. Now, as I prepare to become a physician assistant, I approach a different cliff in my life, but the same principles of preparation, practice, commitment, and confidence still apply.

After identifying my goal of becoming a PA, I availed myself of opportunities to explore the healthcare field and advance my education. One of my most rewarding experiences was volunteering at the People's Health Clinic in Park City, Utah, where uninsured individuals receive free care. My responsibilities included taking patients' vitals and escorting them to exam rooms, and I experienced great satisfaction when patients expressed their gratitude for the clinic and for my services. Volunteering at this clinic solidified my desire to provide healthcare services and use my talents and skills to give back to my community.

I have always had a strong desire to make a difference in the world, and I found a way to achieve this personal goal seven years ago. After touring a homeless shelter called The Road Home, I discovered that the residents' most requested item was new socks, so I established the non-profit organization, Stoked On Socks. We collect new pairs of socks and donate them to those in need, proving again that one person can make a difference in the lives of others. When I complete my PA training and join this profession, I will continue to make a difference.

In my current position as a respiratory assistant, I enjoy working with patients. I once fitted a woman with a CPAP mask and educated her about obstructive sleep apnea and the use of the CPAP machine. She described her sleep problems and the negative impact on her life, and I reassured her that the doctor had ordered this course of treatment because he believed the therapy would help her. A few days later, she excitedly reported that she was sleeping better and no longer needed naps during the day. This was one of many experiences where I would have preferred becoming more involved in the patient's continued treatment. My current position as a respiratory assistant allows me significant autonomy while working with patients, and should I need additional guidance, a respiratory therapist is always just a phone call away. As a PA, I will work in an autonomous environment where I will fulfill my desire to diagnose, treat, and provide follow-up care.

Providing healthcare services in times of distress is a valuable contribution. As a youth group volunteer, I helped provide services when another adult leader fell and split his chin. We were hours away from the nearest hospital, but we were fortunate to have a doctor with us who had brought his suture kit. The doctor cleaned the wound and sutured the man's chin. He asked if I would like to put a few sutures in, and with the patient's permission, I proceeded. Although I appreciated being involved, I wanted to be the one doing all of the sutures, treating the wound, and removing the sutures after healing had taken place. As a PA, I will have the skills and knowledge necessary to respond to emergencies and remain involved throughout the treatment and follow-up process.

With every step of my preparation to serve as a PA, my passion and desire increases. I have shadowed numerous physician assistants and enjoyed watching their interactions with patients. While shadowing a PA in neurology, I watched as she and the doctor reviewed a patient's brain scan and pointed out small irregularities. In a recent anatomy course, I had thoroughly studied the identical portions of the brain and the areas of the body that are affected by them. I instantly applied this classroom knowledge to the real world of healthcare, and it was exhilarating to make that connection.

I know that my career as a PA will be exciting and fulfilling. Attending a physician assistant program will be extremely intense, but the principles I used to achieve the skill level of a professional snowboarder will also apply to this aspect of my life. I will be determined, dedicated, and committed to my goal of becoming the best PA I can possibly be.

Essay II (893 words)

I was born in a small industrial city in Russia. My father was a cardiovascular surgeon and my mother is a Feldsher (equivalent of Physician Assistant (PA) in the US). My father left our family when I was 2 years old, and I never met him again. But I was always told that he is a hero, because he saves people's lives. I remember my mom working hard on two jobs to give me the best education she could. Thus, I was a busy kid, and at the age of 9 I had graduated from musical school in class piano, took English lessons in one of the private schools, dance classes, and all the while still attending my elementary school. Since my mother was busy all the time, I was taken care of mostly by my grandmother who lived with us. We were very close to each other. Then, when I was a teenager, she suffered a stroke. She survived, but after that was sick for a year. It was a painful time for both my mother and myself. I was 15, and now it was I who helped take care of my nana every day after I got back from school. I saw her in pain, not being able to eat, or use the bathroom without help. That year of grief absolutely opened my eyes on what I wanted to do with my life—I wanted to help people.

During my final year of high school, I volunteered at the Skin and Venereal Diseases Hospital where my mother worked. I remember seeing her with the patients and how she would ask them to smile. Later she explained it as a trick, "If you ask them to smile then they feel much better after doing that than after taking the medicine." I observed and helped doctors and nurses perform procedures on patients. I learned medical terminology, how to collect lab specimens, and obtain vital signs. I walked patients to the tests, helped them with dressing up, taking baths, and skin care. But the most valuable thing that I learned is to keep your heart open with patients who suffer from pain and disease. They need to be not only treated with procedures and pills, but also to be heard and emotionally supported.

At 17 years old, I moved to the bigger city and the capital of the country—Moscow. It was a time of new opportunities and choosing my career direction. My oldest cousin who lived there and worked in television had influenced me to become a journalist. I studied journalism at Moscow State Humanitarian University for 5 years. This opportunity gave me invaluable experience with the skills of gathering, analyzing, and delivering information and putting it into a format that is understood by others. I learned how to verify facts, to be trustworthy with sensitive information, to be able to relate well to a wide variety of people, and to adapt to constantly changing circumstances. But soon I started to realize this was not what I dreamed about doing with my life. By working as a journalist I was serving people with information, but I wanted not just to serve them, but to help them—big difference! I decided to take a break in my life and find my true path.

At 22, I participated in the International Student Exchange Program. I came to the United States and decided to start all over again. I always knew that I wanted to work with people, to make them feel better. Therefore, I pursued a Bachelors Degree in Biomolecular Sciences—the first stepping-stone in my medical career. During my first year of study I had to become proficient in English very quickly, thus my grades suffered in the beginning. Yet, after a lot of hard work, my English improved and studying became easier. Soon, I became a Dean's List student and was awarded scholarships for academic achievement.

During this time, I was able to shadow a PA in the Emergency Department. I was impressed by his work with critically ill patients and resolving acute emergencies. I have seen and followed patients from their admission through discharge from the hospital.

My other shadowing experience was with an Orthopaedic PA from Connecticut Children's Medical Center. I observed him working with patients during regular office exams and also in the Operating Room where he and the rest of the surgery team performed limb lengthening and deformity correction.

Presently, I work as an Emergency Medical Technician in the Emergency Department. This experience is teaching me how to work under extreme conditions of stress. I am also always interested to learn from observing the PAs and MDs who work there, asking them to explain x-rays and CT scan images. I want to become a PA because of a long path that started with my mom and the example she gave me. Like her, I want to enjoy the direct contact with patients and most of all to be able to help people who are in serious need. I am 26 now, married, and a stepmother myself to three beautiful girls. I am ready to spend my life dedicated to helping other families like mine and to achieving a life/work balance. I know that the best way to accomplish both of these goals is to become a PA.

Essay 12 (864 words)

"Rand missus?" The boy held out his tiny grimy hands, eagerly, hopefully. Most striking was the smaller child standing next to him, a gaping hole extending up from his split upper lip. I handed the boy the change I had, knowing it could do little to improve their situation, but wanting to do something. Their hopeful, expectant faces created a poignant image that remains with me, even now, 15 years later. It was during this trip to the war ravaged capital of Mozambique, as a young exchange student studying in South Africa, that I first became truly mindful of the physical consequences of poverty. I felt quite helpless at that time and wished I could do more for them. My brief encounter with them, and similar experiences while in South Africa, made me realize that I didn't want to be helpless. I wanted to make an impact in the lives of those around me. Specifically, I decided that I wanted to pursue a career path, where I could contribute to the health and well being of my community.

Returning from my studies abroad, I changed my major to Anthropology. I knew that I wanted to go into some sort of health field, and felt strongly that understanding people and the cultural context in which they exist would be a good start. I also completed all of the pre-requisites for applying to medical school. Following graduation, rather than medical school, I chose to obtain a graduate degree in public health at the University of Utah. This proved to be a natural complement to my studies in anthropology and a very rewarding experience. I really felt like I had found my niche and hoped it would provide me the opportunity to make a positive contribution to the community.

I was fortunate to get a job with the Utah Department of Health, Office of Epidemiology, in the sexually transmitted disease (STD) surveillance program. My responsibilities included working collaboratively with a variety of health care professionals, including medical providers, public health nurses and social workers to ensure that all those testing positive for reportable STDs were properly treated and partner follow-up was conducted. My co-worker and I met with and interviewed minors with STDs in detention facilities and drug treatment centers across the Wasatch Front. We also developed an educational presentation on STDs and their prevention which we presented at various facilities across the state. Seeing the frequency of STDs in specific youth populations, I wrote and was awarded a CDC grant to assess the magnitude of the problem in Utah. Through this grant, we were able to actively screen for STDs and pregnancy in over a thousand at-risk youth in detention facilities, drug treatment centers, and a homeless youth clinic. We also wrote and administered a survey to those we tested, in order to better understand the types of high risk behaviors that were increasing the risk of infection in this population. This also provided an opportunity to meet with and discuss individually, strategies to help these teens stay safe and healthy in the future. At times, our interactions were emotional and challenging, but I always felt that we were able to make a positive difference in the lives of these youth.

My career as an epidemiologist was cut short due to personal health problems. In retrospect I believe these health issues were a mixed blessing for two reasons. First, I had the opportunity to be a patient, a role that I'll admit to not relishing. I experienced the relief and gratitude a patient feels when treated with dignity, sincere concern and respect. I also was the recipient of care that was lacking in these qualities. These experiences had a profound impact on my view of the responsibility health care providers have to their patients. I understand that healing a patient physically is not always possible. However, I do believe that the best care is always delivered compassionately, respectfully and takes into consideration the individual's entire health picture. Secondly, the time away from my work as an epidemiologist allowed for significant introspection as to whether I felt I was accomplishing my personal and professional goals. From this I realized that what I really wanted was to work more closely with patients than what I was able to as an epidemiologist

As my health improved and I began to assess the options available to me, I quickly came to the conclusion that becoming a physician assistant would allow me to fulfill my goals. I believe that my life thus far has really prepared me for this profession. The role the physician assistant plays in health care delivery is perfectly suited to both the innate and acquired skills I possess. I believe that both my anthropological and public health training along with the maturity and commitment I posses as a non-traditional student will help me succeed as a PA student and physician assistant. I know that once I become a physician assistant, my curiosity, ability to actively listen and engage, along with empathy and my sincere desire to serve others will enable me to make a significant and positive impact on the health and well being of my patients.

Essay 13 (520 words)

The Physician Assistant (PA) profession fulfills a unique niche in medicine. The aspects of this career that makes it so interesting and fitting for me are: the team dynamics of working with physicians, nurses, and other health care professionals, the opportunity and flexibility to work in different subspecialty areas, and the ability to spend more time with patients than the supervising physician. I particularly am drawn to the dynamic of collaborating with physicians to ensure quality care is given. The particular aspect of the PA profession I desire is the ability to be trained as a generalist and further the education to a specialty if I desire.

Commitment, resilience, and the skill sets I have developed can only be discussed by referencing my prior experiences. Accepting Teach For America's offer to teach in low-income schools across the country, where I did not know anyone, was pivotal. My level of commitment was tested and approved. I became devoted to helping an underserved population, even though it meant leaving my friends, family, and everything I've known behind. The resilience of teaching came in the ninety-hour work weeks, driving students home, and relentless pursuit of success of my students. The best part of the Teach For America opportunity was being challenged with tough circumstances and few resources yet preserving through them to get results. This program and my previous experiences have proven that I am committed to my passions and resilient to persevere through obstacles. Through my experiences I have exemplified my strong interpersonal skills, self-determination, organization, time management, and empathy towards others. My ability to effectively and concisely communicate with the individuals was a vital component to success. Simultaneously, my organization and time management led to my student and athlete's success, which was fueled by my empathy, passion and determination to relentlessly ensure they were reaching their goals.

One thing I am improving upon is my multitasking. In college and high school, I did an impeccable job juggling work, school, athletics, and multiple volunteer activities. However, I never could fully devote to an activity that I felt strongly. Through teaching, I've worked to not stretch myself, which led to great successes with my students.

My involvement working with diverse communities has been a lifelong commitment through teaching, Special Olympics, caring for patients in home care, and assisting women in a battered shelter. I excel in places where I am stretched to creatively and professionally care for individuals different from myself. I am committed to continuing to do so in the PA profession.

Pacific's PA program offers unique and exceptional opportunities to hone my skills in the medical field and provide exceptional healthcare to diverse populations. The opportunities to improve my Spanish and provide international healthcare while in school are two of the ways Pacific will support me in working with diverse populations in the medical profession. Pacific's impeccable reputation to successfully prepare students for success on the boards and beyond is essential for my goal attainment. Thus, this program would help me to not only successfully develop my skills to be a PA but also to thrive into the future within the profession.

Essay 14 (883 words)

Some of us are fortunate enough to have a person enter our life that has such a profound impact that it forever changes the direction of our lives. For me this was my brother-in-law's mother. She had an amazing capacity for giving that was evident from the first time I met her. Judy was a nurse who spent her life dedicated to helping others, ultimately becoming one of the first hospice nurses in northeastern Ohio, working with the Hospice of the Western Reserve. I did not realize the magnitude of her impact on my life until last year when she lost her battle with brain cancer. I was moved to tears as person after person stood up at her funeral and spoke of the positive impact she had on their lives and the comfort she provided. It was at this moment that my life changed forever.

I had known for some time I had to make a change. My entire career had been spent working in the corporate world where all that matters is the bottom line. I needed to find a way to help others and, more importantly, to make a difference. In the months following Judy's funeral I struggled to find the correct fit. Soon after I had my first experience with a physician assistant and everything became clear. After suffering a stress fracture in my leg I was referred to an orthopedist. The PA that did my initial assessment was truly amazing. She spent a great deal of time explaining my injury and discussing my x-ray and MRI, covering all the structures involved. I immediately began investigating the PA profession and became more excited the more I learned. The teamwork, the collaboration, and the autonomy all caught my attention. These were all aspects of working that I not only enjoyed, but also excelled at during my 20 years working in information technology. After months of considering a career change I knew I wanted to become a PA.

Once I made the decision to pursue a new career as a PA I pursued as much knowledge and exposure as I could. I immediately contacted the Ohio Association of Physician Assistants to obtain a list of PAs to shadow. I was fortunate to be put in contact with a great PA working in Orthopedics. Shadowing Sarah allowed me to see first hand the positive impact PAs have on their patients. I spent a good deal of time with her and really got to know her patients. I found myself taking an interest in Sarah's patients' care and looked forward to seeing them again and following their progress. The PA shadowing was such a positive experience I wanted to do more. Unfortunately with 20 years of IT experience I found it difficult to find a patient-centered position. I decided to volunteer at a local hospital in the trauma unit. The volunteer position has allowed me to interact with patients and gain insight into the hospital environment. Just seeing the joy brought to a patient by the simple act of getting a warm blanket or a glass of water has provided me with a sense of purpose.

The biggest obstacle in my path is my early academic performance. Despite taking the college prep curriculum in high school, I was not challenged academically. I graduated near the top of my class with minimal amount of work. Once I started college it became apparent this approach would not be successful. I lacked the necessary study skills but was too proud to reach out for help. Prior to my second year, my parents divorced and I was forced to move out on my own. It seemed that overnight my focus shifted from being simply a student to needing to support myself and pay rent. I struggled to balance school with working enough to meet my basic expenses. My school attendance and grades both suffered. The low point came when I was dismissed from Ohio State University. This was the wakeup I desperately needed. I used this time to reflect and focus on getting my life together. I began a job at a computer store, then worked my way into the corporate IT world where I was promoted several times and moved into positions with increasing responsibility. When I returned to school I was more mature and ready to succeed. I had learned to manage my time, set priorities, and most importantly to ask for help when I need it. My grades over the past several years reflect this maturity and focus. I have rededicated myself since returning to complete my PA prerequisites, making the necessary sacrifices to maintain a 4.0 GPA, all while still working full time.

While I may have a nontraditional background, my experiences and adversities have prepared me well for this next, challenging stage in my life. I have the high level of commitment and dedication necessary to be successful. Most importantly I have the desire and passion to not just help others but to make a difference in their lives. I have been asked numerous times if it is hard to give up the lucrative career I built in IT to return to school. The answer is always a simple "no," because I now realize this is what I am meant to do.

Essay 15 (860 words)

At 17 my doctor diagnosed me with Scheuermann's kyphoscoliosis and a spinal curvature of 90 degrees. I underwent a full thoracic-lumbar spinal fusion from vertebrae C3 to L4 at Shriners Hospital. From the moment I was extubated in the operating room and through the week of re-learning to walk, the nurses, surgeons, and medical staff gave me comfort and hope in a time of unbearable pain. When initially looking at the X-Rays with new hardware screwed into my spine, I was instantly intrigued how one procedure could change my posture and my life. Through the course of my recovery, I dreamed of the possibility I too could change lives through medicine. Many experiences influenced my desire to choose the Physician Assistant (PA) profession as my means of helping people through healthcare.

Although I was unprepared to excel at such a competitive level when I began college, my knowledge flourished after gaining healthcare experience at a level one trauma hospital. After my sophomore year, I shadowed Medical Doctors (MD) and inadvertently the PAs at Tampa General Hospital (TGH) to explore and learn about medical professions. I was unaware of the PAs' role but impressed I could not distinguish between the knowledge and technique of the MDs and PAs. While rounding with the critical care team, I noticed the PAs had more time to assess and connect with their patients. One of the PAs was so personable to her patients that many times patients preferred to see her instead of their doctor. The PAs taught me various treatments and pathologies they manage day to day such as tracheostomies and sepsis. They also exemplified their responsibilities when responding to a code blue and managing the airway of a patient. I now understand the important role of the members of the PA-MD team model and know that the more personal patient interaction of the PA is the perfect profession for me.

After deciding to become a PA, I aspired to expose myself to many fields in the medical arena to prepare for the diversity of the profession. I began this journey by working in clinical research with the anesthesiology and surgery departments at TGH and was intuitively involved in the academic side of medicine. Our team collaborated with the University of South Florida College of Medicine and focused on innovative surgical techniques, novel burn dressings, and varied analgesic regimens; leading to numerous publications. My patient interaction with research linked patient care to the constantly changing world of medicine. In an effort to provide the most recent and effective care to patients, being involved in clinical research is important to me as a future PA.

I continued my mission by volunteering as an emergency medical responder at Florida State University. I learned and demonstrated the urgency and alertness one must possess when arriving at an emergency. My skills were put to the test when I arrived at the scene of an unconscious male who fell off his skateboard resulting in a large laceration to his head. Arriving and assessing the scene to distinguish between a medical or trauma emergency and acting accordingly made these types of calls suspenseful and challenging. This experience will help me with decision making as a PA when handling stressful cases and making critical diagnoses.

My view of medicine expanded beyond my comfortable borders after traveling to the mountains of Buff Bay Jamaica with a diverse team of medical professionals. In a span of ten days we diagnosed and treated over 700 Jamaicans who otherwise had no access to healthcare. Prior to going on this trip the need in underprivileged countries carried no relevance in my life. This trip opened my eyes to the reality that people all over the world live where little to no health education or resources exists everyday.. The overwhelming gratuity and constant joy of the Jamaican people, despite limited material possessions made every day at clinic inspirational. I returned to America realizing that my motivation to become a PA was not one of self gain but of service to those in need.

Finally, I expanded my role at TGH by working as a patient care technician on the neuro-surgery floor. This job led me to care for diverse patients ranging from stroke to psychiatric patients and the unique opportunity to care for patients recovering from spinal fusion surgery. . My firsthand experience was invaluable for connecting with patients who were often doubtful or anxious about their recovery from spine surgery... This opportunity gave a sense of comfort and hope to my patients that believed no one else understood what they were going through; a quality I hope to display as a PA.

My preparation for becoming a PA has allowed me to view medicine through multiple lenses. I have seen that despite the diverse environments where healthcare occurs, the mission remains the same: providing a tangible way to love and heal the hurting. My long term goals as a PA are twofold: working in surgery and actively participating in local and international medical missions. If given the opportunity, I am confident my clinical experience has afforded me maturity, drive, and focus to excel in PA school.

Essay 16 (769 words)

The journey began at a mere four years old. The dream and goal were set by eight. The sacrifice, focus, and dedication that would be necessary were realized by ten. Great success came by sixteen and a bittersweet feeling by 23.

"Lub-dub, lub-dub, lub-dub"; I could feel my heart beat. I could faintly hear "U-S-A, U-S-A, go Danielle!" echoing from the bleachers as time counted down in the championship fight. "Three, two, one, ding"; I had become the Pan American Champion at 16 years old. These are the sounds and feelings that have filled my soul since 8 years old and have stayed the same; training after training, kick after kick, year after year, through the past fifteen years of taekwondo competitions. All the missed football games, dances, and sleep, combined with long drives and extra training, paid off. Eventually, they led me to a training partnership at the 2008 Beijing Olympics, a spot on two national teams, and 5th place at the 2009 World Championships in Taekwondo. More importantly, I walked away with skills and intangible life experiences which, paired with my parent's unparalleled love, have made me into the person I am today and have given me a clear vision for the future.

Discovering the greatness of having a team, the joys of travel abroad, and the importance of taking care of your body, are three of the greatest gifts that taekwondo has given me. Despite taekwondo being an individual sport, our team is the backbone of our individual success. We feed off each other's energy, athletic knowledge, and motivation. We all have different upbringings, values, and personalities, but love and support each other like a second family.

In addition to my friends and teammates locally, travel to over 15 countries has introduced me to different cultures and great people around the globe. Eating local foods and experiencing local traditions have made me appreciate every way of life. Thanks to my travels, I have made good friends in Guatemala, Denmark, and Mexico.

All of my travels have been meaningful. However, my most impactful trip was to Brazil. I remember driving from the airport to the hotel. We passed mountainsides of adobe-like one-bedroom homes with dirt floors, no running water, and children running barefoot through the streets. For the first time in my life, I felt powerless, sadness, and a rejuvenated desire to help.

As an athlete, understanding your body and training it to achieve maximum efficiency is key for longevity. It is incredible how our bodies can withstand strenuous exercise and how each body system functions together to maintain optimal performance. Throughout my years as an athlete, cutting weight and pushing myself to the max has taught me the best ways to fuel, strengthen, heal, and rest my body. All of these experiences have helped me to better understand myself and the type of work I would enjoy. But, the daunting question still remained; what did I want to be when I "grew up"?

I knew I enjoyed my science classes. I knew that the intricate physiology of the human body amazed me and that I found fulfillment in helping people from all backgrounds. However, it was not until mid-junior year, when a fellow classmate and I were conversing about our future career goals, that I first heard of a Physician Assistant. He proceeded to explain to me what a PA did and the path to become one. Suddenly, a feeling of relief came over me; "Wow that sounds perfect!"

In the following months I shadowed several Physician Assistants. A PA at Miami Children's Hospital became my mentor. Not only did she let me shadow her, but I got to accompany her to hospital meetings. She encouraged me to start working with patients. Now, after 9 months as an orthopedic tech assistant, my passion to help people has only grown.

Although I lack extensive direct patient experience, if given the opportunity, I will work diligently to become an important member of the healthcare team. I am prepared for a rigorous course of study and excited for all the practical applications. As a future Physician Assistant, I look forward to working both independently and collaboratively with supervising physicians in a challenging environment. I want to provide a better quality of life for my patients. As my dad, a speech and language pathologist in nursing homes, once told me, "No matter how long you have been working, never forget to treat every patient and person with purpose and compassion." These are the words I live by as I embark on my new journey to becoming a successful Physician Assistant.

Essay 17 (803 words)

Jambo! Welcome to Kenya—my native land. Strolling through the vast streets of Africa, a few right and left turns takes you to the baseball fields of Kisumu Elementary

School. It is the perfect day, with the sunshine giving enough warmth as to rid the wind chill, for the title game against the rival elementary school. Thus far, at the end of the 3rd quarter, both schools are tied and I am the last player up to bat. With fierce determination and a bat in my hands, I studied the thrower with a glance that spoke louder than words. Two fast pitches and he had knocked me off my base. Yet even when the pitcher held the ball in his hand with the confidence to settle my team's fate, I resolutely maintained my conviction of winning the game. I swung the bat vigorously as the ball came to me and...and the ball flew to the sky. We won; my team had won!

Contemplating back to that memory I am reminded of just how immensely different the achievements of a child versus those of an adult are. As a child, I was overwhelmed by a mere baseball game win. However, today my ambitions are to prepare myself for a new, more challenging goal; to become a physician assistant.

At the tender age of 8, I arrived to the United States along with my family to pursue the "American Dream". Only those who are immigrants can comprehend the adversities of adjusting to a new language, a new atmosphere and a whole new lifestyle. The first day of 5th grade was the longest day of my life. I still remember how I didn't go to the bathroom for the entire day because none of the kids understood me when I asked where the "loo" was. Although, I eventually learned to grow into this new lifestyle and, while I will never forget my background, I learned to adapt to my new environment. Thankfully, along with the hardships, came rewards. Being in the "land of opportunity," meant that now I had the opportunity to strive towards any goal I could possibly conceive of.

As I went on to high school and college, my desire to be a PA has been continually reinforced. I was able to gain firsthand experience in patient care quite early in my college years. One of the most satisfying volunteer experiences I had was when I was an emergency medical technician at Montclair University's EMS for over a year. In that time, I learned that medicine is nothing like I had thought in the past. I still remember, only a few months into my training, I saw my first critical patient. "Lub dub, lub dub, lub dub". The man had Ischaemic heart disease. I found that he died just minutes after he was discharged to the ER. He just laid there—pale, empty, lifeless—just laid there. Although this transpired at least twenty times on episodes of House M.D., actually seeing first-hand this situation was a really life changing experience for me.

Forthwith, the satisfaction of being an EMT diminished considerably. I realized that I tended to patients for particular ailments but then I was to never see them. I would begin to wonder; what happened to them; will the Ketoacidotic patient that I took care of last year live to see today? Perhaps I would never know, though I sincerely wish I did. As a physician assistant, I would be able to provide comprehensive care to my patients and be available to them for on-going consultation, which is one of the essential reasons why I aspire to become a PA.

One of the most interesting experiences I encountered during my undergraduate college was taking part in research. Though I certainly enjoyed classroom learning and all it had to offer, I excelled when it came to hands-on learning. Research with Dr. Adams on inhibition of SinV Virus, responsible for the Sindbis fever, prevalent in Kenya and other parts of Africa, was truly intriguing so much that I devoted more time into research then I had ever thought possible. The one aspect of medical research that still amazes me is knowing that I, a mere college biology student, understands something that no one has grasped yet. Research is what I can take pride in, though monotonous and tedious, I feel as if I am accomplishing something great, even if it may be miniscule in the grand scheme of things.

Being a physician assistant would give me the opportunity to fuse all my interests and career goals together. While research is invaluable to the path of discovery, volunteering as an EMT has shown me that patient care is where I really belong since I would be able to fulfill my long-term career goal best that way.

Essay 18 (339 words)

Several years ago, I had the opportunity to reevaluate my life plans. I realized I wanted to begin a career in the medical field, and entered a medical assisting program. During the training, I learned of various medical careers, and became captivated with the physician assistant profession. I discovered it is one of the few medical professions that not only allows involvement in patient care, but also in diagnosis and treatment.

At present, I work in a family practice office as a back office medical assistant and scribe. This means that I also have the opportunity to work alongside the doctor during each office visit. I add history, diagnoses, physical exam details and treatment plans to the office visit note while the doctor is performing the exam. Meanwhile, I also scan the electronic medical record for information that would be important to that particular visit. For example, when the doctor is considering certain medications that may affect kidney function, I look to ensure the patient has no diminished kidney function on recent lab results. I question the patient and doctor for clarification, and I propose diagnostic tests or treatments for the doctor's consideration. Observing the doctor's ability to determine when a firm hand or compassionate hand is needed has also been extremely enlightening.

I have also had the occasion to see the healthcare field from a patient's perspective. A recent diagnosis of simultaneous ovarian cancer and endometrial cancer has allowed me to see the difference a compassionate caregiver can make to a patient who is in the midst of a serious diagnosis. It has also taught me the value of early diagnosis and treatment.

I currently live in a medically underserved rural area, and understand many of the challenges of such an area. In particular, I am reminded of one elderly diabetic patient who could not afford to drive the few miles to pick up his insulin at the office where I worked. I brought it to his tiny house on my way home. That day, he also asked me for information on diabetic diets; I brought a book to him the next day.

I would prefer to work in family practice as a physician assistant where I could care for patients with varied conditions and backgrounds. I look forward to future challenges and rewards of a lifelong career as a physician assistant.

Essay 19 (1346 words)

"A PA helped save my daughter's life" exclaimed my co-worker Christy. She detailed how the persistence and advocacy of a PA at the ER had been instrumental in diagnosing her daughter with Kawasaki syndrome. As she spoke, I was struck—yet again—by the dedication of this PA; not unlike that of the many other PAs I had contacted in prior months. Though I had been exploring the profession for some time already, it was this defining moment that truly cemented my desire to become a PA.

Growing up outside Bombay, India, my late grandfather had been our town's first doctor; I grew up hearing stories of his love for people and medicine. My grandmother—who suffered a stroke and diabetes—let me to "help" her take insulin shots and medication. Though I was young, these experiences left a strong impression; it was during this time my love of service and healthcare was born.

Growing up in India was a wonderful experience; I learned to interact and live with people of diverse perspectives, cultures, languages and religions. In March 1993, due to ongoing religious rifts, a string of bombs were set off in downtown Bombay. My father's office building was a target; he was trapped for hours before being rescued. Though he suffered only minor injuries, my family was shaken to its core; we immigrated to Canada shortly thereafter.

In Canada, my father was unable to find a job and succumbed to depression and alcoholism. I started working at 15, to help support my mother and younger brother. Though far from ideal, this situation instilled in me excellent time management skills, and a determination to excel. I learned to balance paid work with strong academics and community service. This included volunteer positions at an animal shelter, a sexual and domestic violence hotline, a local hospital, an opera house, and with local environmental groups. Working at the crisis hotline and at the hospital, I realized my true desire was to serve people through healthcare—though I was still unsure of the route I would take.

When accepted to the University of Toronto, I made the difficult decision to continue living at home and supporting my family. Since my decision made me ineligible to receive financial aid, I took on a second job to fund my education. This was a crippling period in my life: emotionally, physically, financially and academically. Despite a strong desire to excel, and an inherent love of learning, I simply did not have the time or the means to demonstrate my academic ability. Coping with my father's disease—and his increasing verbal and physical outbursts—eroded our family finances and all sense of stability. A heavy work schedule, combined with the increased financial burden of education and a competitive academic environment, meant I could not perform at a level that reflected my true academic abilities. Though dropping out of school would have alleviated much stress, I persisted, determined to graduate in good standing, in my chosen field. Though it was the most challenging time of my life, it taught me maturity, adaptability, and most of all, perseverance. I graduated in good standing in 2006, and moved to Texas shortly after.

In 2007 I began work at Cogenics, as part of team that provided molecular biology services to a wide range of clients. The technical and logistical challenges of the job were enjoyable; as was the opportunity to expand on knowledge acquired in university. In 2009, I moved to Biotics Research Corporation (BRC), a respected nutraceutical company that manufactured over a 100 unique dietary supplements. Working at BRC was a tremendous growing experience. As the only Quality Assurance (QA) Coordinator, I supervised a team of 8 QA Associates, as well as acted as a liaison between the Board of Directors and company-wide QA activity. In this fast-paced environment, I learnt crisis management, how to identify and solve unique problems, and most of all, how to effectively work in high stress situations while maintaining my composure and the integrity of my role. The health-related aspects of this job strongly rekindled my desire to work in healthcare; I knew without doubt, that a future profession based on a medical model of education was my goal.

Shortly after I began work at BRC in 2009, my husband was treated for an eye injury by a PA at our local ER. I was impressed with her depth of knowledge, calm demeanor and the ease with which she worked alongside the doctor to treat my husband. She was happy to tell me about her journey into the PA profession; that very night began my quest into understanding the profession more fully. I joined the AAPA, and contacted as many PAs as possible. In the many phone and e-mail conversations that ensued, two similarities stood out—all loved their chosen profession and the team-oriented nature of their jobs—both were traits I strongly valued in any future profession. In shadowing five PAs, I was amazed at the range and complexity of specialties they practice in—from the ICU to cardiovascular surgery—and also at the unique relationship that exist between each PA and supervising physician. It was also during this time I met Christy, and experienced the defining moment that led to this application.

I quit my job in June 2010, and returned to school full-time; I wanted to prove my academic capability and become a more competitive PA candidate. Since then I have completed 42 hours in PA pre-requisites with a 4.0 GPA. I also volunteer in the community: as an adult "English as a Second Language" (ESL) teacher; at Houston Hospice; and most recently at Omega House.

As an adult ESL teacher in an underserved community, I develop curriculum and teach adults to speak and write English. All of my students are immigrants, who—as I once did—cope with various levels of cultural isolation. Being able to empathize with their situation has helped me not only be a teacher, but a life-coach and cheerleader of sorts. I am proud to say that with my help, many have dramatically improved their language skills; some have even gone on to find jobs or complete their GEDs—goals they never thought possible.

At Houston Hospice, I have the honor and privilege of interacting with patients in the final chapter of their lives. Learning to deal with death in medicine was a challenge. Here, I learnt that being a good care-giver means more than administering treatments—it means offering empathy and comfort as well. It saddens me that PAs are still unable to practice in this area of medicine; if given the opportunity, I hope to one day be part of the growing PA movement that is trying this.

While at Houston Hospice, a lead nurse recommended I volunteer at Omega House, where she had previously been Director of Nursing. Omega House is a residential hospice for people in the late stages of HIV/AIDS; volunteers contribute almost 70% of patient care. Here, I have had the opportunity to serve with patients in many ways: by socializing and interacting with them; cooking meals, changing clothes and diapers; helping feed, bathe and attend to personal hygiene; as well helping nurses chart daily progress, remove catheters and administer medication. Both hospice positions have given me a deep

sense of fulfillment, and deepened my longing to be able to serve and treat patients in a greater capacity.

I want to be a PA because I want to be part of a growing profession that is hands-on, practical, challenging and constantly evolving. Working with supervising physicians means exciting opportunities to acquire new skills and knowledge and the ability to practice in more than one area of healthcare. With my strong love of learning, a genuine desire to serve patients and the skills acquired through my life experiences, I feel that I am a strong candidate for the PA profession. If given the opportunity, I also hope to contribute to the PA community by being an advocate for the profession, and by helping educate future generations of PAs.

Essay 20 (856 words)

Some events alter the course of your life and drive you towards a clear goal. At the age of eleven, my friends and I were playing soccer when my friend fell and split his forehead on a rock. In a fraction of a second, blood drenched his whole face and I leapt into action, tending to my friend who was in a state of panic. Despite my own rattled nerves, I pulled out my handkerchief and applied pressure to his wound—a response that was second nature after having observed my mother, a nurse, do the same thing dozens of times. I instructed my friends to call the nurse while I assured him that he would be fine. I felt his nerves begin to calm, and by the time the nurses arrived, my uniform was soaked in blood. They continued to apply pressure to keep him from bleeding to death before he safely reached the ER. From that day forward, my clear and driving passion was medicine. I witnessed firsthand how practicing medicine was not only about prescribing medication or performing surgery but also about caring for people and applying information that could ultimately save lives.

My passion for medicine was deepened when a car accident hospitalized my mother my freshman year of college. During that time, I ended up paying more attention to my recovering mother and my struggling family, working full-time at Whole Foods Market to support my family. My grades suffered, serving as the wakeup call that made me realize that failing to perform my best helped no one and led me to develop better self-management under adverse circumstances. I learned to prioritize my coursework and proudly graduated with a 3.26 grade point average.

Two years ago, tragedy reared its ugly head again when my mother was diagnosed with saddle pulmonary embolism and was admitted at Beth Israel Hospital for two weeks. Our family was grief-stricken at the thought of losing our mother, yet nearly every visit we found her chatting good-naturedly with her PA. They developed a friendship, and I saw what a difference the PA made not only in caring for my mother's physical health but for her mental health as well. The way she accompanied my mother's every step until her recovery triggered my decision to pursue a career as a physician assistant.

My desire to become a PA was enhanced by my research during my senior year of college with a fellow classmate under the guidance of Dr. Mande Holford. Our research focused on Solid Phase Peptide Synthesis of Teretoxins snails and their characterization through HPLC and mass spectrometry. Even more than our findings, we gained valuable lessons on teamwork, diligence, and patience despite setbacks along the way. I was fascinated by the potential of snail toxins to alleviate chronic pain in HIV and cancer patients, and my interest in HIV patients caused me to search for ways to contribute to their well-being. I found the perfect opportunity to join two medical trips in regions severely affected by the HIV epidemic: the African nation of Tanzania and La Ceiba, Honduras. From my first trip, I worked in a rehabilitation center for HIV/AIDS orphans where I met a teary eyed three-year-old boy named Winner, a HIV infected orphan. From the time I first picked him up, it was clear to me that, more than medicine, this boy was desperately in need of love and affection. The highlight of every day was seeing Winner run to me with his arms wide open, and I will always remember the impact I was able to have on one child's life through my service.

Thus inspired, I sought out more ways to make a difference and a classmate and I gathered hospital supplies, including 100 HIV test kits and lancets, and purchased gloves and alcohol pads. We helped test patients for HIV, a project that called on the knowledge and skills I acquired during my clinical rotations for the medical technology program. One of the most heartbreaking tasks I performed was informing an individual that he tested positive, but providing the peace of mind and prevention counseling to many men and women who tested negative gave me hope and left me with a great sense of accomplishment and a desire to do even more.

Wanting to learn more about the profession, I shadowed a PA and observed her as she diagnosed her patients' conditions and determined the course of treatment. Every consultation was an educational exchange where she learned more about the patient and their symptoms and educated them on preventative care, including proper nutrition and home-based exercise protocol. Her dedication to her patients only reinforced my decision to become a PA, as I was constantly reminded of the care my mother had received two years prior.

From my friend's encounter with a rock to coping with my mother's illness to my experiences in the field, I know that becoming a PA will allow me to lead a life of significance where I will directly impact lives and care for those in need. I look forward to taking the next step on this journey.

Essay 21 (812 words)

"One hundred twenty five, one hundred twenty six, one hundred twenty seven," I counted, as I waited for the second hand to reach one minute. The patient's pulse had increased at an alarming speed. As an emergency medical technician (EMT) I was the only certified health care professional in the gymnasium when the woman started experiencing chest pains and dizziness. She refused further medical attention and expressed the desire to drive home, but my instincts told me that she needed further medical attention. The gym owner left it to my discretion as to whether to call my squad for backup, and I knew the woman was trying to squelch her fear by refusing further medical treatment. I knew what I had to do.

I sat with the woman as I called the ambulance, and she began to relax as I explained how I could help her as an EMT-B. My psychology degree comes in handy as I address patients' emotional concerns, while my tactical emergency medical skills help me tend to patients' symptoms. On this occasion I presented the information to my fellow EMTs and relayed the status to the charge nurse when we arrived at the hospital via ambulance. I was glad to utilize my skill set and instincts to help this woman receive the care that she needed, and I long to impact many more people as a physician assistant (PA).

I experienced the life of a PA when I shadowed at Monmouth Medical Center. Despite their policy to only allow graduate students to shadow PAs, as an undergraduate student I knew I had to be persistent in order to attain my goals. My dedication paid off and I found myself shadowing physician assistants in the emergency department and volunteering in departments across the hospital. In my work with patients I witnessed the role of communication skills and bedside manner; my duties included serving as a liaison between patients and their health care team, relaying the patients' questions and concerns. Despite not providing physical care, I knew I had impacted the lives of patients and their families simply by giving them respect and attention. I am eager to marry my compassionate nature with the application of medical knowledge that PAs employ as they diagnose and treat patients.

Shadowing PAs in the ER and later at Seaview Orthopedics showed me the in-depth nature of their patient interactions. Not only do PAs order and interpret tests but they spend time with patients to thoroughly explain the results. Physician assistants also provide reassurance when a patient shows signs of unease; I remember a patient I encountered when shadowing Nadine, an orthopedic PA. He had suffered a complex injury that required a complex treatment plan, and Nadine took the initiative to draw a picture of his injury and what it would look like after treatment was completed, explaining the treatment and the recovery process. Despite her numerous responsibilities, Nadine never left a patient until they were satisfied with their treatment and all their questions were answered, and her approach taught me to show compassion to each individual rather than treating a patient like a chart number. Just as I immediately came to the aid of the woman in the gym, I will do the same with my future patients.

While shadowing various physician assistants I noted their relative autonomy and how when the PAs consulted with the physicians, their education and skills complimented the training of the physician. Observing this reminded me of the way a well-trained EMT crew works together seamlessly. Being aware of each other's abilities allows us to work fluidly while treating patients, and on emergency calls we anticipate what a fellow EMT might need or how our actions may impact them. My time as an EMT has prepared me to recognize the limits of my abilities and the importance of communicating with those with more medical authority.

I believe that physician assistants are so in tune with physicians because of the medical education credits they accumulate. The constant evolution of the medical field forces them to keep current with advances in medicine and technology. One PA explained to me that she had just earned credits toward her license by taking a quiz based on recent medical journals about developments across several areas of medicine. I am excited by the constant learning required, understanding that we must stay attuned to developments in the medical field. Through my determination, compassion, and experience I am confident that I will be an outstanding physician assistant, effective not only through my hands but through my heart as well. The gratification I gain from each encounter with the health care field has given me a taste of the incredible rewards I will receive during my career. I look forward to embarking on the next step of this journey to become a caring and healing physician assistant.

Essay 22 (522 words)

Giving up or getting discouraged by obstacles is simply not in my nature. The adversities I have faced have shaped my character and motivated me to keep moving forward at every turn. My decision to forge a new path as a physician assistant was not a change of career I took lightly, but once I set my mind to it, I never had a moment's hesitation.

It was the biggest decision of my life to leave a successful career in the music industry, the only career I knew and one to which I had devoted years of my life. My volunteer experience and years of work as an EMT in inner-city Atlanta left no doubt in my mind that this was the right decision. When you finally find something that you love and know is right, you will move mountains to get there. Moving those mountains requires patience and perseverance, and I have employed them both to get where I am. While my grades from over twenty years ago do not accurately represent my abilities, my more recent science coursework and efforts in my daily healthcare work better reflect my potential. I have always risen to the occasion, never shying away from difficult circumstances, and I feel these characteristics will benefit me as I embark on this next stage of my career.

My efforts over the past year and a half have moved me much closer to my ultimate goal of becoming a physician assistant. I have been working at a family practice owned by a husband and wife physician team with two PA's. It is a wonderful learning environment as the office handles everything from general medicine to urgent care. They are fantastic teachers who involve their team in the treatment of every patient so as to provide the best care possible. I am grateful for the opportunities and support they have given me, and I especially appreciate the opportunity to work as part of a true team. Whether in my career as a music manager, as an EMT or now as an MA, I have always thrived in a team environment. This is one of the many facets of the PA profession that appeal to me.

In addition to my demanding hours working at a busy family practice I continue to volunteer at the free clinic, one of my favorite places to be. It is inspiring to be a part of a team that provides such critical services to those who cannot afford care. It is also a challenging environment as approximately 90% of the patients speak Spanish and my Spanish is limited, but this experience has strengthened my commitment to my studies in Spanish.

While I wish I had found my passion for this path earlier in my life, I feel fortunate to have discovered it at all, recognizing that many people spend their entire lives searching for their true calling. Since beginning this quest towards a career as a PA I have gained substantially more knowledge, focus and wisdom—qualities that will serve me well and will be a tremendous assent on my journey towards becoming a PA.

Essay 23 (654 words)

I have known I was meant for a career in medicine ever since an incident in the summer of 1990. Some friends and I were playing a little rough when my friend Doris's toenail was accidentally ripped off. No adults were around, so despite the profuse amount of blood and Doris's hysterical crying, I knew we had to do something. My fear and nerves were no match for my intense desire to help Doris, so using a first aid kit from my parents' closet, I cleaned her wound and applied bandaging until her mom could get her to the doctor. Doris will probably always remember that day as traumatic, but for me, it was the day that I realized that practicing medicine was not just about taking vital signs and giving medication, but about giving patients the best care possible and peace of mind about their condition. I was hooked and knew that a career in medicine was my goal.

Upon my undergraduate graduation, I became an HIV/AIDS case manager in Camden, NJ where I worked closely with clients, families, social services, and medical professionals to coordinate services for people dealing with myriad life challenges. It was an invaluable experience that taught me to be empathetic and objective while focusing on the task at hand; I got up every morning ready to improve the health and wellbeing of my clients through care, compassion and respect. After serving as a case manager, I taught special needs students, not only providing daily instruction for them but tending to their basic medical needs as well. Because of my character and my passion for medicine, the school administration was confident in my ability to handle minor scrapes and bruises. Even parents of the most medically fragile students were comfortable with my first aid CPR training and my ability to react swiftly to emergencies.

While I gained valuable experience from serving as a HIV/AIDS case manager and from working with special needs students, the most significant aspect of both positions was the deep awareness I gained of the healthcare disparities between the affluent and the underprivileged. In communities where needs are the greatest, educational resources and quality of healthcare are the weakest. I knew I wanted to make a difference by pursuing a career supporting physicians serving urban communities.

I have both innate and acquired skills that will make me a successful physician assistant, recognizing that the requirements go far beyond empathy and awareness of societal injustices. In other professional roles, I have been deemed a highly competent leader, organized and assertive but never aggressive. I understand the competitiveness of the PA applicant pool, however, as a non-traditional student I bring maturity, preparation and confidence to my cohort. Since completing my bachelor's degree in psychology, I have completed upper-level science courses that have broadened my awareness and will help prepare me for a PA program. For example, in a recent genetics class, I researched the genetic disorder Osteogenesis Imperfecta and learned about the delicate process a healthcare team undertakes when a mother with this condition delivers a baby.

I am prepared for a rigorous course of study and for the practical experience that will lead me to a successful career as a physician assistant. I know what the job entails, as I have had the opportunity to observe physician assistants conducting physical exams, diagnosing and treating illnesses, ordering and reading tests, counseling patients on preventive care, writing prescriptions, and empowering patients. I have seen how physician assistants must act as independent thinkers and doers while also consulting closely with supervising physicians, and I understand the role that they play in a healthcare team. Moreover, my background as a case manager and public school teacher has prepared me to serve high-risk populations, which aligns with my goal of serving in urban communities. I look forward to giving as much back to the profession as I know it will give me.

Essay 24 (607 words)

After graduating from the University of Utah in 2003 with a degree in political science, I began my career as a lobbyist for public higher education in the great state of Utah. This was my dream job, or so I initially thought. I will always be grateful for the invaluable people skills I honed while lobbying on the Hill, not to mention the thicker skin I grew, but I was just not satisfied professionally. For several years following graduation I found myself pursuing numerous employment opportunities from being a dorm parent for troubled youth in rural New Hampshire to working as a legal assistant in a law office. I even thought about furthering my education in professional counseling or public administration and signed up for graduate classes. Even though each of these paths complimented my strengths and sparked my interest, none of them were quite the right fit. None evoked my true passion...until six years ago (enter choir: "Hallelujah! Hallelujah!"), when I discovered how rewarding and fulfilling being a physician assistant could be. I was hooked.

My metamorphosis began as a medical assistant in a large orthopedic practice where I worked with several physician assistants and their doctors. Though the doctors were impressive, it was the physician assistants who showed me the rewards of providing quality health care through patience, compassion and patient-centered approach. I was particularly inspired by the additional time the PAs spent with each patient, educating them on their ailment and explaining treatment options in layman's terms. This orthopedic group also treats the underserved migrant community in South Florida. I found this part of the practice especially rewarding, as I was able add medical terminology to my Spanish vocabulary while witnessing patient gratitude that was both humbling and motivating. Interacting with these patients made me long to be able to care for and treat them myself as a physician assistant.

Throughout my journey I have been fortunate to have exceptional mentors who encouraged me on my path towards becoming a physician assistant. I was advised to explore several areas of medicine, so in addition to orthopedics I worked and volunteered in dermatology, family medicine and urgent care. Even during the recession, when my hours were cut and jobs were scarce, I continued shadowing physician assistants and volunteered as a medical assistant on a regular basis. These very special practitioners instilled in me that the goal of every physician assistant is to ensure patient education, which in turn results in patient compliance and effective treatment. Thanks to them, my understanding of the role of a physician assistant is clearly defined as an extended care provider who delivers superior treatment. As an integral part of a health care team, I will assume the role of patient advocate and ensure that their needs are always met or exceeded.

I have spent the last six years preparing for this application process. Having found my perfect fit, I returned to school with a focus and drive like never before. Unlike my undergraduate coursework, where grades took a back seat to leadership and advocacy opportunities, I have dedicated myself to my academic preparation for the PA program and I am confident in my ability to perform in a demanding academic and clinical setting.

From my undergraduate activities in student development, leadership and advocacy, to writing and recording a hit song for ESPN, I am confident that I will add to the diversity and distinction of the 2013 entering class. I will fulfill the high standards of excellence commensurate with the physician assistant profession and will give back as much to the medical community as I know it will give me.

Essay 25 (495 words)

I am applying to the George Washington University Physician Assistant Program in order to advance my clinical knowledge and to gain the skills necessary to provide a higher level of patient care. Upon completion of the PA program, I plan to provide care to service-members wounded in combat and HIV/AIDS patients living in poverty, two under-served groups with which I am very familiar. I also plan to continue my research work as a Principal Investigator for clinical trials.

I earned a Bachelor of Science degree in Zoology and a Master of Science degree in Preventive Medicine from Ohio State University. The Preventive Medicine program focused on community and population health, biostatistics, and epidemiology. During college, I was employed as an Emergency Medical Technician (EMT) with the Ohio State University Emergency Medical Services and at the University Medical Center Emergency Department. For my master's thesis, I worked with the Ohio Department of Health, analyzing survey-question responses and the associated risk of HIV infection utilizing multiple-regression analyses.

After receiving my masters from Ohio State, I worked as a Clinical Data Analyst for a 350-bed hospital in Reno, Nevada, providing support to clinicians and hospital administrators in the identification of best practices and other quality improvement initiatives. I was promoted to Business Manager of Emergency, Trauma, and Surgical Services and was responsible for the financial health of each of these departments. I served in this position for two years.

For the last eleven years, I have worked in the pharmaceutical and medical device industries, managing clinical trials as a Clinical Research Associate. I have worked in many therapeutic areas: cardiovascular devices; infectious diseases including HIV and Hepatitis; endocrinology; pain management; autoimmune disorders like Crohn's Disease and Rheumatoid Arthritis; pediatrics for Type I Diabetes and vaccine clinical trials; etc.

I have been involved with community service beginning in my teens as a volunteer firefighter and EMT in my rural Ohio town. While living in Nevada, I was a volunteer technical search and rescue technician and EMT with the Washoe County (Reno) Sheriff's Office. Eighteen months ago, I enlisted in the US Army as a combat medic and currently serve with the US Army Reserve 75th Combat Support Hospital. I am a squad leader and responsible for organizing continuing education for the combat medics in my unit. I volunteer as a Community Outreach Representative with the Wounded Warrior Project. I am also training as an Honor Guard member, to serve at the funerals of service-members who have made the ultimate sacrifice.

All of my life experiences have lead me to this point and have created within me the passion and desire to provide my community and country with a higher level of care as a Physician Assistant. GW's commitment to community service and its diverse urban environment drew me to this program. As a graduate of GW's PA program, I will be able to serve my country and community by providing them with the level of care they truly need.

Essay 26 (852 words)

While volunteering at Second Wind, a riding stable for people with disabilities, I experienced profound joy at hearing an autistic child on horseback say her first word and seeing the ecstatic expression on a man's face when he realized that, even though he was paralyzed, he could still ride. As a physician assistant, I will have the opportunity and the privilege to influence people's lives positively every day.

My experiences at Second Wind and my love of science inspired me to major in medical technology. This healthcare-related field allowed me to study nearly every branch of science, and it seemed to be an ideal fit. I loved the coursework, and I especially enjoyed the focus on human pathology. My first job as a medical technologist was in a very small clinic. I enjoyed many aspects of my work, but I did not feel challenged and longed to utilize all my skills and training. I spent much of my time performing phlebotomy, and most of our samples were sent to a larger laboratory for testing. To prevent stagnation of my education and knowledge, I transferred to a larger lab.

I quickly realized that utilizing a more complex skill set was not enough for me to feel fulfilled. After a period of intensive introspection, I realized I need a career that includes direct interaction with patients. When the phlebotomists need assistance, I am eager to help them and to interact with patients. From providing therapy to autistic children to volunteering at Planned Parenthood, the highlights of my experiences have always been my direct interactions with patients. Although there is a patient connected with every lab sample, there is no face or personality for me to associate with it. I am an important member of the healthcare team, but I don't feel like a participant in individual patient care.

The best part of my first job was forming relationships with patients. As I prepared to draw blood from an elderly gentleman, I noticed that he had visited a doctor in another clinic that morning. When I informed him he could have had his blood drawn there instead of driving all the way across town, his response was, "I know that, but you won't screw it up." His words let me know how important it was for him to have someone he trusted draw his blood, and I felt honored to be that person. As a physician assistant, I will always be mindful that a patient's trust is an essential component of optimal healthcare.

I met another patient who came in regularly to have her Coumadin levels monitored. On her first visit, I asked her to be seated in the draw chair, and she burst into tears. She had recently undergone knee replacement surgery, was unable to tolerate her pain medication, and could not bend her knee enough to sit in a chair. The simple solution was to place a stool in front of the chair so she could keep her leg straight while sitting. On every visit thereafter, I made sure there was a stool ready for her, and on her final visit, she gave me a card to thank me for my patience and compassion. What I considered a simple act to provide comfort meant a great deal to this woman, and she confirmed that simple acts of caring make a big difference to a patient. My enthusiasm for my current work stems from the opportunity to employ my critical thinking and troubleshooting skills. My most important responsibility is to report accurate results for every test. Recently, I reviewed a patient's critically low calcium level, which had been normal just the previous day. It was obvious to me that this result could not be accurate and was not reported. These analytical skills and attention to detail will be invaluable when diagnosing a patient.

My participation in a Wilderness First Responder course through NOLS provided insights into comprehensive patient care. In this course, we learned to properly assess a patient, collect necessary history, provide treatment using few resources, and complete SOAP notes. To date, I have not utilized this knowledge in my field of clinical lab practice, but the classes made me aware of how much more I enjoy caring for the patient as a whole as opposed to performing strictly diagnostic testing.

My background as a medical technologist will give me an advantage as a PA. In addition to my familiarity with multitasking, I have a strong grasp of interpreting laboratory results, and I understand how these results are derived. I will know when to utilize a particular test method or identify potentially inaccurate results. Since most diagnoses utilize lab results in some form, my background will serve me well on a daily basis. As I reflect on the knowledge and skills gained from previous jobs, I feel especially well suited to a career as a physician assistant. I will be able to incorporate my critical thinking ability, my love of science, and my desire to care for individual patients as I pursue what I am convinced is the perfect career path for me.

Essay 27 (850 words)

As I regained consciousness, I wiped the blood from my eyes to see my mother standing over me. I was in the back seat of my best friend's rusted '67 Mustang that had collided with an ancient oak tree on a winding dirt road a mile from my home. My mother had been called to the accident site, not as the parent of her sixteen year-old injured son, but as an Emergency Medical Technician (EMT) with the volunteer service she and my father helped start just a few years prior. This accident would serve as the initial inspiration for a journey through many roles in healthcare, ultimately leading to my desire to become a PA.

I was rushed to the local Emergency Department (ED) with a ten-inch laceration to my scalp, and it was here that I had my first encounter with a physician assistant. He was a former Navy Corpsman like my father, and after the attending physician ruled out injury to my cervical spine the PA assumed responsibility for my care—an arduous and lengthy task of debridement and suturing. He showed concern for my pain and the emotions that were consuming my mother, periodically stopping to reassure us that although the injury appeared severe, with ample suturing and time it would heal without any permanent damage. As often happens with encounters during dramatic times, his calming nature and professionalism remains etched in my mind 25 years later.

Wanting to gain exposure to the medical field, during breaks from my freshman year of college I volunteered as a firefighter and EMT in my rural Ohio hometown and ended up working with the same PA who had cared for me two years prior. He always showed a keen interest in my education and experience as I transferred patient care over to the ED staff, asking me questions about the patient and taking time to answer my questions about diagnoses and treatments. His mentorship leads me to hope to do the same for future aspiring PAs.

During the remainder of my undergraduate and graduate years at Ohio State, I worked fulltime at the university Emergency Medical Services (EMS) and Medical Center ED as an EMT-Advanced. I thrived in the fast-paced environment of a Level I Trauma Center, fine-tuned my skills as an EMT, and came to know PAs and PA students rotating through the ED and Trauma Service. They were always enthusiastic and eager to document history and physicals, were skilled at performing procedures, and interacted in a meaningful way with all patients regardless of ailment or socio-economic status. In addition to the experience gained, my graduate program in preventive medicine equipped me with the knowledge and skills to promote health through risk-reduction, disease identification and preventive medicine. I have employed these skills throughout my medical career and know that they will be key to my work as a physician assistant.

Having had meaningful clinical and educational experiences, I learned about the business of healthcare as business manager of Emergency, Trauma and Surgical Services for the largest hospital in Reno, Nevada where I balanced the compassion of caregiving with the business of healthcare and supplemented a physician shortage in a remote community with the skills and expertise of PAs. While I already held PAs in high regard, my respect for PAs only increased as I witnessed their dedication to providing uncompromised patient care in a high-pressure environment.

I spent the next eleven years managing clinical trials in the pharmaceutical and medical device industries, interacting with physicians, nurses, and PAs on a daily basis. During this time I discovered that it was the PA in the medical practice who routinely consented the subjects for the clinical trial; the PA has the knowledge to answer the subjects' questions about the risks and benefits of the study medication as well as the patience and time to do so, providing an enormous service to the healthcare community in facilitating these trials.

After turning forty during the deadliest year of US military involvement in the Middle East, my focus turned to my lifelong goal of military service to my country. Refusing to live my life with any regret, and passing up officer commission, I enlisted in the US Army in order to serve as a combat medic. At the age of 41, I began basic training and the most rewarding and challenging eight months of my life. I am currently assigned to the 75th Combat Support Hospital where I work as part of a cohesive team of physicians, nurses, physician assistants and medics. The physician assistants in my unit have taken on a mentor the medics, inspiring us to preserve the lives of wounded soldiers on the battlefield. It has by far been the most powerful chapter of my life.

All of my experiences have culminated in a desire to advance my knowledge of the human condition and to gain the skills to aid my fellow man; these experiences have fueled my desire to become a physician assistant and I will give back as much to the profession as I know it will give me.

Essay 28 (649 words)

The last few years have been a time for me to reflect, review my career objectives, and plan for change. I want a medical career with a promising future and direct involvement with people. My future career must meet my need for continuing education, provide an opportunity for change, and utilize my past life experiences, training, and skills.

The physician associate profession meets that criteria, and the viability of the physician assistant profession is without question. The creation of a national healthcare system that demands affordable healthcare will only intensify the need for PA's, and indicators suggest that this profession will grow throughout the next decade and beyond. I still have twenty to twenty-five working years ahead of me, and I want my next profession to be one that will offer both challenge and opportunity.

The role of a physician assistant goes beyond the treatment of symptoms and encompasses a deeper level of knowledge, compassion, and continuous learning. Most effective healthcare professionals have empathy for their patients, along with the required skills and expertise, but a physician assistant makes a greater contribution to society, and I am eager to fill that role. I look forward to making a contribution to my community and society.

For approximately fifteen years, I have been practicing as a chiropractic physician, and I have established a reputation for providing high-quality care to my patients. I have communicated and coordinated care with primary care physicians and specialists in meeting patient needs. Most referrals to my practice come from other healthcare providers, and I attribute their confidence in me to my abilities as a team player and my understanding that a multidisciplinary approach is sometimes necessary. Having a family with small children made my decision to change careers a difficult one, but I feel it is best for my family and for our future. Years of adjusting patients, including the strenuous activity associated with the physical therapy and chiropractic techniques I utilize in my practice, are beginning to take a toll on my body. I enjoy what I do, but my job is physically hard on me, and I don't want to lose my passion for helping people because of it.

The other compelling reason for choosing the physician assistant career is that the profession has made tremendous advancements in the medical field, and it has worked to improve the future of the profession. I do not have those feelings about the chiropractic profession. We seem to have so many differing philosophies and agendas that, instead of growing stronger, we have alienated ourselves from one another. My goal is to participate in a profession that will continue to grow, become an integral part of our healthcare system, and develop the essential tools and resources necessary to best serve public healthcare needs.

During my undergraduate years, I had to cope with my father's alcoholism and the effect it had on our family, and my academic performance suffered because of that. My grades in Chiropractic College, however, reflect my level of maturity and my commitment to succeed. Some of my extracurricular activities, from elementary school through college, include my interest in music and my ability to play the Bouzouki, an ethnic Greek instrument. I formed a professional band that performed weekends at festivals, weddings, baptisms, and parties. To help finance my undergraduate education, I also owned and operated a hot dog concession stand during the summer months, and I worked at numerous jobs with a variety of people. These experiences greatly enhanced my communication and social skills.

An effective physician assistant collaborates with supervising physicians while maintaining independence and nurturing a good rapport with patients. My commitment to becoming a PA is unequivocal. During my career, I acquired the analytical, communication, and time management skills that will help me become a truly competent physician assistant, and I am confident that I will be an asset to the profession.

Essay 29 (758 words)

"Do it for the kids" is the motto of St. Jude Children's Research Hospital's Up 'til Dawn organization. This simple, yet powerful motto kept me motivated as I faced the daunting challenge of being a full-time student, full-time residence hall director, and committed leader of Illinois College's new organization, Up 'til Dawn. This organization raises funds and awareness for the children of St. Jude Children's Research Hospital. As the Executive Director of this organization, it was my responsibility to act as the liaison between Illinois College and St. Jude Children's Research Hospital. It was a collaborative effort which united faculty and staff with the students for one cause. Without the help and support of an outstanding team of committee chairs and committee members, we would not have been able to raise over $22,000 for the hospital. We truly "did it for the kids!"

I enrolled in Illinois College as a freshman during the fall of 2006. By the end of freshman year, I had decided to pursue a career as a physician assistant. My interest began when I was treated by a physician assistant who was a kind and knowledgeable healthcare professional. I wanted to have the ability to provide the highest quality patient care possible, while maintaining a calm and friendly atmosphere. Working as a physician assistant will allow me to work autonomously in providing patient care, while still giving me the opportunity to consult with a supervising physician on the more challenging and complex cases. I am pleased to know that as a physician assistant, countless opportunities are available as new interests arise. Regrettably, my first year at Illinois College was not spent giving adequate attention to my studies, and consequently, my grades suffered for that. I used this as a learning experience. I knew that if I was serious about being a physician assistant, I would need to buckle down to achieve my goal. While participating in many on campus groups, I was able to continuously increase my GPA through a combination of hard work, better time management and prioritizing my career goals. As I continued to challenge myself my senior year, I not only was able to take an 8 credit hour EMT-B course in addition to taking 19 credit hours at Illinois College for my undergraduate degree, but I was able to make the Dean's List both Fall and Spring semesters.

Just months after graduating from Illinois College and completing my undergraduate degree, I earned my EMT-B license. With a burning desire to work as a physician assistant, I continued to seek additional healthcare knowledge and experience. In an attempt to quench this yearning, I enrolled in an accelerated EMT-Paramedic course. Since July 2010, I have worked for LifeStar Ambulance in Jacksonville, IL gaining over 3,500 hours of direct patient care experience. Working in EMS has helped me gain a much better appreciation for the important roles that various team members play in providing quality patient care. Every day I go to work, I realize the impact we, the healthcare team, have on our patients' lives. There is a satisfaction felt deep inside when I make a difference in the lives of my patients and this fuels my passion to do more. With my experience working in EMS and working with other healthcare professionals, it is evident that physician assistants play an invaluable role in the healthcare system and I intend to become one of the best.

Through my experiences, I have successfully developed skills that will allow me to succeed as a physician assistant. Through my involvement in Up 'til Dawn and working as a hall director, I have gained valuable experience with groups of diverse individuals, as we establish common goals. Working as a paramedic has been beneficial and allowed me to expand on the skills I learned at Illinois College as I work within a healthcare team. Together, the care that we provide in collaboration with the many healthcare professionals at the hospital has proven how beneficial being a team player can be.

I have dedicated the past five years of my life preparing myself for the role as a physician assistant. My community service and educational pursuits have allowed me to mature, gain additional healthcare experience, and demonstrate my deep compassion for making a positive impact on the lives of others. I possess the dedication, desire, and determination needed to be successful in the physician assistant program. By successfully completing the physician assistant program, I will have the skills and knowledge required to provide outstanding care to my patients.

Essay 30 (505 words)

My desire to pursue a career in medicine as a physician's assistant is a product of my professional and personal background, my work ethic, and my desire to have a positive impact on the lives of others. For the past 15 years I have practiced chiropractic medicine, which has provided me with invaluable clinical experience in treating those ailments that respond to chiropractic modalities. Initially, it was the most rewarding endeavor of my life—the culmination of years of difficult schooling, clinical hours and hard work. However, with that same clinical experience and professional growth, I became increasingly frustrated with the limitations of chiropractic practice and felt that something was missing. I was searching for a common thread in medicine, a more comprehensive vantage point that would allow me to treat a broader spectrum of medical conditions so as to be of greater help to my patients. In my view, I was seeing just a piece of the puzzle, and not the entire solution.

Moreover, it was frustrating to have been educated in the medical model but to lack prescriptive authority. Ultimately, while I have enormous respect for chiropractic medicine as a means to an end, I became professionally unfulfilled and dissatisfied. It was this yearning to be a more complete healthcare practitioner that led me to pursue a career as a physician's assistant.

Despite these philosophical concerns about my chosen profession, it was a recent life-altering experience that ultimately fueled my passion to make the change: my mother was diagnosed with lung cancer. While following the course of my mother's disease I had the opportunity to meet her doctors and interact with them on a professional level. Their dedication and tireless pursuit of the best possible treatment inspired me and re-ignited my own desire to pursue something more fulfilling. During this time, I became immersed in obtaining the best care possible for my mother, exhaustively researching the drug regimens and protocols best suited for her. Though it may sound a bit lofty, this personal mission further reinforced my belief that practicing medicine was my purpose in life.

In addition to my personal inspiration, I believe I have the right sets of experience to be successful in this field. Having practiced chiropractic medicine in inner city neighborhoods for the majority of my career, I have developed patience, understanding, and compassion from working with people of different cultures and ethnicities—traits that are essential when working as a physician's assistant.

I feel that my passion, dedication, clinical experience and maturity make me an excellent candidate for a program of your caliber. As an adult in my mid-forties and as a licensed chiropractic physician, I fully understand the commitment and stamina needed to meet the challenges of medicine and I possess the intellectual requirements and critical thinking skills needed to be an outstanding physician's assistant. I look forward to giving back as much as I know I will gain from the program and from the profession, and I respectfully thank you for your consideration of my candidacy.

Essay 31 (748 words)

In the trauma unit, I approached a new patient to obtain his consent for our Traumatic Brain Injury study. The patient wanted to go to the restroom, and I assisted him so he would not fall. Back in bed, he complained that he had not eaten lunch, so I found the duty nurse who told him he had already had his lunch and left the room. Becoming very upset, the patient started to cry and confided that his family, including his adult daughters and attorney brother, had abandoned him. Realizing his depression, I listened to him, encouraged him to be strong, and suggested he see a psychiatrist. After we talked for fifteen minutes, he felt better and appreciated my attention and respect. This experience greatly reinforced my desire to become a clinician and a director of patient care.

With my training and background as a clinician in China, it is now my dream to continue to direct patient care in the United States. I attended the Clinical Program at Xavier University Medical School where I did a fifteen-month U. S. clinical clerkship and sub-internship. During my training, I learned about the physician assistant profession and, for some of my rotations, I followed a PA when the physician was not available. The broad medical knowledge, accurate diagnosis, and sharp clinical skills of one PA impressed me enormously, and I admired his dedication to his patients and his satisfaction with his career. Later, when I worked as a medical assistant at a dermatology surgical center, I met another PA. After working with her, I gained an appreciation for the potential autonomy and opportunities for critical thinking that this career has to offer. As I learned more about the role of a PA, I realized this would be a better career goal for me than that of a physician. Not only can I take full advantage of my broad medical knowledge and clinical skills, but I can also fulfill a strong desire to continue my personal growth in the clinical field while having more time to fulfill my family responsibilities.

Having made that decision, I have devoted myself to preparing for PA school. I joined the AAPA, strived to obtain high GRE scores, took prerequisite courses or refreshers, and was able to shadow various specialty PAs at Parkland Hospital, St. Paul Hospital, and Children's Hospital. I learned that PAs have a unique role wherein they focus on an array of specialties under the supervision of a medical doctor but also work autonomously to assist physicians. Understanding the current challenges of the PA profession and the increasing demand for PAs, I am very passionate and excited about the opportunity to become a PA. Working as a volunteer at the West Side Clinic, a major volunteer community clinic providing limited primary care for the indigent and uninsured adults of Collin County, has provided me with another unique experience in this special clinical setting and reminds me of a homeless shelter in Atlanta where I once volunteered. These experiences will help me deal with similar situations in my future clinical practice.

The PA profession is very challenging, but I have a lot to offer, and my hands-on clinical experience in the United States will be a big advantage. As a clinical study coordinator for about three years, I often supervise junior study coordinators or mentor medical students with their research and heavy daily workload. This gives me the opportunity to use my excellent communication and interpersonal skills, provide efficient time management, and set priorities. I learned to be a team player and a team leader. Four years of teaching experience in medical school in China and in my U.S college has honed my excellent interpersonal skills. With more than three years of work experience in the information technology field, I am comfortable applying my computer skills within the medical field. In addition to my full-time job, and to improve my English as much as possible, I also participate in the Toastmasters Club. Interacting with my fellow members helps me to fine-tune my listening and speaking abilities, and these vital skills help me better understand and serve my patients.

My desire and commitment to becoming a physician assistant is so strong that I will not allow any obstacles to deter my progress. I intend to make the most of every opportunity to achieve this goal, and I look forward to bringing my strong motivation, reliability, interpersonal skills, and capacity for hard work to this program.

Essay 32 (620 words)

From my experience, positive outcomes are the most rewarding when achieved through hard work and perseverance. Through my trials of attempting to gain admission to physician assistant school, I have learned that preparation and time management skills are assets of achievement. In order to further my knowledge and better myself as a health care professional, I chose to re-take many of my science classes and continued to shadow physicians and physician assistants to learn more about the process that guides the decisions of those who operate in the health care field. I recently became a member of the Student American Academy of Physicians Assistants and the American Academy of Surgical Physician Assistants, associations that fuel my passion for the profession and through which I stay current in the field.

It is often through challenging circumstances that we are able to focus on what matters most to us. I recently suffered a tragic loss when both my parents passed away within three months of each other. Through their illnesses I became deeply involved in the care of both my parents, resulting in a renewed passion for the art of medicine. As the eldest of three children, I was called upon to make critical decisions related to my parents' care, a responsibility that made me acutely aware of the ethical trials that come with end of life decisions. With a heavy heart, I honored my mother's wishes to not be resuscitated while the rest of my family pushed desperately for a different route. My father suffered from a staph infection that caused his body to succumb to sepsis; despite my knowledge of the evils of sepsis, I honored my father's wishes of aggressive care in spite of the devastating ordeal he had just been through. When my father's condition deteriorated, I assisted the short-staffed team with CPR until more personnel could arrive. While obviously a heart wrenching time, I knew I had to maintain a positive and professional medical mindset.

Choosing my field of study was a simple decision, as I have been interested in medicine from a young age. While in high school I joined our local fire department and took EMT classes. As a rural department, our emergency services were the only medical services available for a thirty-mile radius, and this deep involvement sparked my dedication to helping others. As an adult, I was eager to pursue my paramedic licensure, and since completing the program I have maintained my EMT-B license and practiced emergency medicine.

I currently work at a Level I Trauma Center where I collaborate with physicians, physician assistants and other health care personnel on a daily basis. I have witnessed that the practice of health care is a team effort, and I have seen how communication and trust are key to solid team relationships. I have also gained experience as a technician in the surgical intensive care and burn intensive care units, roles that allowed me to examine labs, communicate with providers, and perform simple procedures like wound VAC care, assisting with skin grafts, and burn care.

I have the motivation, education, maturity and medical experience—including rehabilitation, wound care, emergency medicine, and critical care—to succeed in my pursuit of this degree and to become an outstanding physician assistant. I have the skills to assist and manage a team that will provide the best possible outcome for patients and their families, and I will apply a positive outlook to the intensive training that I will receive in the program. I look forward to taking the next step towards achieving my dream of becoming a physician assistant, bettering myself while embracing the education that will allow me to have a positive impact on the lives of others.

Essay 33 (838 words)

I am one of the lucky ones; the ones who know what they want to do with their lives. Today, more than ever, I know I want to become a physician assistant. The year 2009 had ups and downs that gave me insight about what I can do and gave me the wisdom to do it. My desire to become a physician assistant is inspired by my mom's battles with cancer, my dad's example as a physician in Ecuador, my personal experiences as an immigrant, and through my work serving the healthcare needs of underprivileged communities.

My mom was diagnosed with colon cancer in 2000 at the age of 72, her second time facing this devastating disease. Her disease affected me not only personally but professionally, and my experiences with her treatment inspired me to become a patient advocate. On one occasion, I went with my parents to my mother's doctor appointment and realized the many challenges and misunderstandings they faced. With only limited English skills, they didn't ask questions of the doctors or staff, just nodding and smiling to show respect. Another time, when my mom was receiving chemotherapy treatment, a lady sitting next to her asked for ice in Spanish but nobody understood her. I requested it for her and proceeded to translate a booklet of information for her. The gratitude she felt was only outweighed by my mother's pride watching me help this patient. Sadly, my mom lost her battle with cancer in 2002 but her healthcare experience, her courage and her words of inspiration made me realize that I wanted to pursue my dream of becoming a physician assistant.

The seed of working in medicine was planted long before my mother's illness, however. Growing up in Ecuador, I marveled at how caring and perceptive my father was with his patients and their families. I remember my dad showing me an amethyst and a quartz rock given to him as a symbol of appreciation and payment from a miner whose leg my dad had saved. I was so proud of my dad not only for saving the man's leg but for his openness to accepting these rocks as a form of payment. I began to picture myself following in his footsteps to help improve the lives of others.

After moving to the US, to gain more experience in the healthcare field I worked at a community health clinic in San Diego, where my language skills were invaluable. I remember assisting a Spanish speaking grandmother who suffered from diabetes. While conducting a health education session, I realized she had no idea what the physician had told her. Immediately, I called the doctor and interpreted for both. It is easy to take something as basic as understanding what someone else is telling you for granted, and I realized what a privilege it is to help someone understand her diagnosis and treatment. It also made me realize the deficiencies in a system where not every patient can understand what is happening to them, and further fueled my desire to advocate for patients as a PA.

Though I was accepted to a graduate PA program in 2009, a slippage in my grades prevented me from continuing. But over my two semesters there I learned a great deal, not only academically but about myself as well. I know what an intensive program looks and feels like; I struggled and overcame most of my academic challenges and my practical skills allowed me to demonstrate my strengths and interpersonal skills. I assisted with the HINI vaccination clinic where we served 2,000 residents of various ethnic backgrounds, and I performed physical examinations on the elderly at nursing homes. However, the program was not structured in a way that promoted student learning, and 75% of the class was placed on academic probation at the end of the second semester. The program lacked any support including tutors, and though I tried to receive help from instructors, their time was limited as they were working professionals. While preparing to reapply, I have learned new techniques to succeed in an academically intensive program. My passion for helping patients live healthier lives has not faltered, and I am committed now more than ever to becoming a physician assistant. I just need a second chance.

My experiences in life professionally and personally have prepared me for a career as a physician assistant. I believe that, like my dad, I have an innate ability to care for people and to help them with their medical care by relating to patients from other cultures and understanding their linguistic and cultural barriers. As a physician assistant I will have the tools to help underprivileged communities and to provide the best care for those in need. I am ready to live up to the challenge of becoming a devoted and successful PA. Roads take twists and turns but I am evermore sure of the path I have chosen. I look forward to giving back to the program as I know I will gain.

Essay 34 (523)

My first shift assignment at the hospital was transporting a patient back to his room. I introduced myself and saw that his left leg had been amputated, a complication of living with diabetes for over thirty-five years. He could not understand why I was willing to serve as a volunteer and he told me how the system had failed him. The center did not process his claims correctly, he explained, and their inefficiency made the process very difficult for him. Eventually, I had to turn my attention to my next assignment, but I promised him I would return. He looked doubtful, and when I did return later, he seemed stunned to see me again. He told me no one ever came back and the staff was constantly changing. As I continued our visits, we developed a friendly relationship. During our final visit, he wished me well and said I would be someone who could make a difference in the healthcare field. His confidence in me made me realize that a career in health care would be the best fit for me, and it strengthened my desire to play a significant role in patient care.

My volunteer efforts brought me into contact with many patients, and I learned to appreciate and value the relationship between patient and healthcare provider. When volunteering at the Elgin Mental Health Center, I spent a great deal of time listening, counseling, and talking with patients, and these interactions were tremendously satisfying for me. Providing community-based counseling and support services that fostered hope, well being, and self-esteem taught me a great deal. I learned the importance of empathy, support, and time spent listening to patients. Assisting patients with their recovery has enabled me to develop effective communication skills, and I have become proficient at teaching and sensitive in demonstrating compassion. It means a great deal to me when I hear patients say, "We can't wait for our next group discussion."

As an undergraduate, eager to provide a voice for those in need, I led various student groups and university departments in organizing programs that expose atrocities threatening the lives of people in many parts of the world. One of these programs was called, "Voices from Darfur," which promoted awareness of one of the most alarming humanitarian crises. I listened to the testimonies describing mental anguish and physical trauma and found it heart wrenching. As I listened to these stories, I became even more committed to the medical field and more passionate about helping others. As a physician assistant, I will work in public health at a significant level of medical intervention, and my heart will be as involved as my mind.

I enjoy direct contact with people in rapidly changing environments. I will welcome the opportunity to work directly with patients in serious need and enjoy using my analytical and time-management skills while drawing upon my community service experience. A career as a physician's assistant is one of the most rewarding in today's society, and I feel strongly that it is my true calling. I am confident I have a great deal to offer to those who need my help.

Essay 35 (828)

Exhausted, I urge myself to do just one more bicep curl. Next to me, a pair of elderly men are discussing test numbers and supplements. It is clear to me that one of them has just been diagnosed with prostate cancer. Immediately, I'm transported to the time I worked in research and the feeling of helplessness I experienced working in academia—this is why I need to be a physician assistant (PA). I could never return to research without being able to treat my patients.

Overcome, I realize that I need to be a PA. I must understand the details of how the body interacts with its environment and why. Moreover, I desire the capacity to address my patient's needs at a level that allows me to diagnose and prescribe treatment for them. At this point in my life, I have exhausted the idea of becoming a doctor, and do not want to spend the money or time earning the title, knowledge, and prestige associated with that career. I, Erin, need to be a PA because it would give me the opportunity to practice medicine and treat my patients in the shortest time possible—meeting my long-held desire to be a health care provider.

My journey has been long and lesson-filled, providing me with a strong foundation in humility, compassion, and empathy. I was born in the "Valley of Sickness" to a man crippled by multiple sclerosis, and a goal-oriented mother. Living in a rural area where people work at fast food restaurants and logging companies, we were surrounded by friends and family who lived on government checks. Accordingly, our loved ones suffered from poor mental and physical health. My family was not spared. My upbringing left me with an understanding of what it feels like to be helpless or "less than," which has been useful in helping me relate to my patients.

My life's mission is to serve those in need, and my thirst for science put me on the pre-medical track. In addition to taking a heavy course load, I worked as a nurse's aid and home health aid. My patients taught me about the value of life and to view the patient as a whole. These lessons helped me gain patient rapport, making me a better care provider. However, my work also taught me that I want to have a career with some level of autonomy, knowledge, and respect. Nursing did not seem to fit that mold, so I ruled it out as an option.

During the summer of my junior year of high school, I went to Ecuador to learn Spanish. Upon my return, I graduated a year early and attended Beloit College. While at Beloit, I studied off campus in Ashland, WI and again in Ecuador to become proficient in Spanish and to improve my understanding of minority populations (Ojibwa Indian and Quichua). These experiences were instructive, because they gave me a perspective on the way people around the world live. They also solidified my desire to work for people in need and to serve them. As a PA, I will recall these experiences and use them to identify with my patients.

Everything was on track, until I got sick during my junior year of college. The diagnosis stifled me, emotionally, not physically, for several years. I changed my focus in life, and decided to attend graduate school because I thought I was a different and lesser person. During my graduate education, I became more independent and confident in my abilities by conducting research in two areas: on methamphetamine consumption among women and epilepsy in Mongolia.

After earning my master's degree, I became a health educator for the health department. I supported the Clean Indoor Air Act by enforcing compliance, researching, creating, and promulgating literature. Also, my team and I cooperated to create and support minority and youth activist groups to reduce the impact of tobacco on the community. While my work was exciting and impactful, it did not "fulfill" me. So I decided to pursue research since it would get me a little closer to medicine.

Working as a research assistant allowed me to gain greater confidence in my work, improve my attention to detail, and increase my independent thinking ability. Most importantly, it allowed me to learn about the PA, MD, and NP profession first hand through discussion and shadowing. Those opportunities taught me that the PA profession is meant for me. From the moment I decided to become a PA, I have committed myself to the preparation for PA school by taking classes, joining PA academies, and reading current PA literature.

My abilities and experiences are uniquely suited for the PA profession. I have spent my life witnessing, working, and researching medicine. This has had a profound effect upon me, not only teaching me about medicine itself, but also imbuing me with a strong sense of empathy and compassion. My curiosity, intelligence and drive to treat the physical and emotional needs of my patients will make me an excellent PA.

Essay 36 (763)

A Ghanaian woman from the remote village of Kwame Danso flashed her hands twice and then held up four fingers indicating to the eye care team that she had lived with this blinded right eye for 24 years. The Unite for Sight team had evaluated this woman's condition earlier at their Charity Eye Clinic outpost and gave her five cedis needed to pay for transportation to the ophthalmologist's home for surgery. Originally, she had developed ptgeryium, which resulted in a corneal cyst and blindness. Through team effort, she received the much-needed surgery to remove the cyst. I'll never forget the woman's expression of joy with her restored vision. This woman had waited a long time as the eye condition did not hurt and she was not aware of Unite for Sight. During my stay in Ghana I worked with a team of local healthcare professionals providing care to patients living in extreme poverty. Every day, our eye clinic team traveled to remote villages on rugged dirt roads to provide eye assessments, care, and glasses to hundreds of patients. Seeing the grateful expressions of those we treated was an extremely moving experience. I felt fortunate to assist in surgeries that sometimes extended late into the night; witnessing the tireless and harmonious efforts of the local health professionals was both exhilarating and inspiring. Because the ophthalmologist had very little time with each patient, I felt a huge sense of responsibility, called upon as I was to dispense medication and provide patient education. I routinely relied on nonverbal communication as my understanding of Twi, their native language, was limited. My immersion into this quality team introduced me to the health care challenges facing developing countries, in particularly educating residents about availability of health care and treatment.

My interest in improving people's quality of life has deep roots. My father, an environmental engineer working at the EPA in Washington, D.C., focuses on maintaining safe drinking water. My mother, a neonatologist, brought me to the hospital many times as I was growing up, giving me early exposure to the health care community. I grew up with a clear view of the rewards, challenges, and sacrifices faced by health professionals.

My interest in patient care was augmented by my experience with Physician Assistants (PAs). In middle school, when I suffered an injury, I was profoundly impacted by my first interaction with a PA, who provided me with excellent emergency room care. After carefully examining my injury, she explained the need for an X-ray and the subsequent need to confer with the radiologist because the image was questionable. Thankfully, I did not have a fracture, but I was left with a very positive opinion of the PA's manner. During a previous emergency room visit for a foot injury, I did not see a PA, had automatic X-rays taken, and after a long wait, briefly spoke to a doctor. The contrast in careful, personable care with appropriate use of resources was immediately clear. More recently, a PA in a dermatology practice put me at ease with her excellent bedside manner. After conferring with the supervising dermatologist, she presented me with an easy-to-understand version of their conversation, making sure I understood the key details. I was so impressed with her that I will be shadowing her later this summer. I also plan to shadow other PAs in different specialties to enhance my understanding of the demands and rewards of my chosen career path.

Working as a full-time undergraduate research intern in the Advanced Imaging Group of the Queensland Brain Institute (QBI) significantly broadened my understanding of health issues, in particularly mental and neurological health challenges. QBI focuses on the diagnosis, treatment, and prevention of neurologic disorders. As the Advanced Imaging Group's only intern, I participated in several research projects using MRI analysis as related to the aging process, dementia, and familial epilepsy, on the published versions of which I'll be listed as a contributor. Realizing that medical care changes with time as new discoveries and treatments come to light, I understand the need to forever be a student, keeping up with new evidence upon which to base practice. With my full time research experience at QBI as a basis, I will review journal articles to provide current information to patients and insight to the hearth care team.

I believe that my background in neuroscience and research, when coupled with my demonstrated commitment to community service and my clear passion for patient care, makes me an excellent candidate for a PA program. I look forward to pursuing a career as a Physician Assistant.

Essay 37 (665 words)

I spent the first twelve years of my childhood living in Pakistan, where the standard of healthcare is marginal. When I was eleven years old, my grandfather suffered a heart attack and had to wait hours at the hospital before a health professional finally assessed his condition. He shared a room with five other patients, and although he pleaded for medical attention, the hospital staff did not respond. Even as a child, I knew that patients deserved better than this. My grandfather passed away later that day, and I will never forget my first exposure to the healthcare system or my resolve that someday I would change it.

My family and I moved to the United States soon after my grandfather's death. As I progressed through elementary and high school, I was confused about which direction to take in the medical field, and I struggled with my options of becoming a doctor, nurse, or physical therapist. None of these career paths seemed right for me, but I knew I wanted to work as part of a team while having the responsibility and autonomy to make my own decisions in patient care.

In 2005, a devastating 7.6 magnitude earthquake hit Pakistan, and the Islamic Relief Foundation requested the help of volunteers. Even though I was enrolled as a full-time college student, I decided to volunteer for ten days in the relief effort. I saw this as an opportunity help others as well as develop my skills as a member of a healthcare team. In the process, I was deeply moved by the devastation caused by the earthquake and its impact on infants, children, adults, and elderly people of all backgrounds and socioeconomic conditions.

I continued my college education after returning from Pakistan, but my mother was diagnosed with a malignant blood disorder in 2007, and my sense of helplessness was overwhelming. During her treatment process, a physician assistant, Aamir Khan, was assigned to her medical team, and I experienced my first contact with this profession. Mr. Kahn and I developed a professional and educational mentorship, and he advised me to enhance my knowledge and skills and begin my healthcare career by working as a nurse technician at a local clinic. While shadowing Mr. Khan in a clinical setting, I learned more about the role of a physician assistant, and this experience confirmed my decision that this would be my future career.

Over the next two years, I continued working as a nurses' aid at the local clinic, working closely with patients, taking vital signs, and collecting short medical histories. We also volunteered and organized free screenings and seminars to educate those within the community and assisted with seminars advocating primary prevention measures such as exercising and smoking cessation. These efforts helped me grow as a healthcare provider and further enhanced my skills and professionalism.

Last year, I applied to several physician assistant programs but was not accepted. I realized I was not up to par with other applicants, and knew I had to strengthen my candidacy. I contacted faculty from each university that had invited me for an interview and asked for their feedback. Acting on their advice, I returned to school in the summer to improve my academic record. I repeated one of my courses and improved my grade from a B to an A. I also worked full time as a certified personal trainer, which gave me even more exposure to direct patient care. My colleagues and I established a volunteer-based community initiative to teach local children the importance of physical exercise and proper nutrition, and I registered as an affiliate member of the American Academy of Physician Assistants. I am proud to have taken advantage of this opportunity to improve myself, both professionally and personally. When my grandfather died, I had a dream of becoming a healthcare provider and making a difference in the lives of others, and I am determined to overcome any future challenges no matter what is required of me.

Essay 38 (1151 words)

I have desired to be a physician assistant literally since the time I discovered what a PA is. Two things set in motion my dream of becoming a PA: First I have had a desire since childhood to help people. The examples shown by both my father and grandfather as ministers were ever present influences on the desperate need of the human heart for healing, as well as the gratification that serving them and helping in the healing process can bring. My heart was stirred to help people-I went on various missions trip with my church to a native American reservation and to Mexico and I witnessed the health needs of the people there, both physically and mentally. The secondary source of inspiration came due to meeting with and being treated by a PA at my doctor's office. Her personable and kind manner set me at ease, and she was truly professional in her work. The initial encounter with that PA caused me to begin to investigate what was involved with becoming a physician's assistant. I shadowed two of the PA's that worked at my doctor's office, as well as a urologist who allowed me to assist in a supervised capacity in several surgeries. Even being given a small taste of the experience of assisting filled me with excitement and passion. The more I researched the role, the more intrigued and challenged I became, to the point of it becoming the professional dream of my life.

The process of learning has always been, and will doubtless continue to be a source of great enjoyment for me. Because good grades had always come easily to me, I misjudged my natural academic strengths when it came to certain college level classes. The mistakes I made related to overloading myself with class and work hours cost me dearly. While I did well as a rule, my math and chemistry class struggles caused me to put my dream on hold and I learned the hard way that in order to succeed academically, I can never make the assumption that a class is easy.

My study focus and efforts required a long hard look, as well as personal scrutiny. After re-evaluating my time management and study techniques, I graduated with my master's degree in counseling psychology. Upon completion of my degree, I was required to pass a difficult exam in order to obtain licensure as a professional counselor, as well as complete 3000 hours of supervised experience. Since that time, I have been employed by Kingwood Pines Hospital for 3 years. While I enjoy interaction with people in their mental and emotional health needs, my dream of becoming a PA never died. In place of the discouragement I had toward becoming a PA, I began to see a strength of combining my ability as a counselor and that of being a PA as one final challenge I was ready to conquer.

With the encouragement of my family and professional colleagues, I felt encouraged to renew my dream of becoming a PA. Equally important to me was proving to myself as well any school that I would attend that I can make good grades and successfully master the math and chemistry courses that stumped me before. Rather than taking short summer courses, as I had before, I carefully and methodically planned my path to success. This meant returning to college and taking over not only the classes with undesirable grades, but also those in which I wanted to have a current and refreshed knowledge. Likewise, the chemistry classes were postponed until after I had spent a semester working individually with a tutor to ensure that I had a firm foundation and comprehension of the subject. Not only have I passed these classes but my grades were superior enough that the dean extended an invitation to join the honors program. My commitment is for this momentum to continue to spur me on to success throughout all remaining courses.

While nobody likes making mistakes or periods of uncertainty, I believe that my experiences have endowed me with more compassion and understanding than I could have had without them. In dealing with patients, I recognize that many of their health problems will likewise result from poor personal choices, but they are in no less need of my compassion. The listening skills and empathy I have cultivated in my practice as a counselor will only serve to embellish the care I hope to provide. Certainly in my dealings with people, I have worked with various personalities many would initially view as challenging or off-putting, but my experience has sharpened my clinical judgment and increased my confidence and assertiveness. My approach will be one of humility, and born of a true appreciation to serve and care for others.

In keeping with this background, I feel that Baylor is the ideal choice for pursuing my education as a PA. After attending an information session, I was struck by the program director's words that he views the program as a finishing school of sorts, where the students are fine polished until they can shine. My desire is to reach my fullest potential, and this statement revealed to me an attitude that the faculty shares in that desire. While at a graduate level, the burden of academic success ultimately rests on my shoulders, it is encouraging to know that instructors will support and motivate me as well.

As a Texas resident, Baylor's name is a familiar one to me. Before learning the formal history of either the school, or the medical facilities, I was introduced to Baylor as a little girl when my grandfather underwent heart surgery in one of its Dallas-based hospitals. In college, I visited a friend at the Waco campus, and the animal lover in me was impressed and excited that they kept bears onsite! Also, as recently as last year, a dear friend of mine faced a life-threatening situation, and it was at another Baylor facility that she received the care she needed to survive.

On an academic level, Baylor impresses me as unparalleled. The ranking in U.S. News and World Report as the nation's ninth leading PA program speaks for itself of the fine education and training its graduates receive. The rigors of a career as a PA demand a comprehensive and meticulous preparation period, and I believe that Baylor will best equip me to meet those demands.

I feel I can flourish in the role of a PA, and if I am fortunate enough to attend Baylor's program, I will do so with the finest of education to support me. My determination has driven me to excel, my previous experiences have taught me that hard work has become my friend, and mediocrity my sworn enemy. The achievement of this goal will propel me to higher personal and professional heights, and truly be the realization of a lifelong dream.

Essay 39 (693 words)

It was a sunny and humid day in the shanty town of Caracas, Venezuela. My surgical gown was damp and my mask stuck to my balmy face. Kids' laughter filled our ears and eased my nerves as they chased each other, barefoot, around the rocky terrain outside of our medical tent. It was the first time I had aided a delivery, let alone one with minimal medical supplies and hours away from a hospital. Ofelia, a young pregnant mother, gripped my hand as I counted down from ten. One last push, and the baby appeared. I helped the doctor drain fluid from his sinuses with a bulb syringe and Ofelia's eyes filled with tears as she heard her son's long awaited first cries. I can still hear her voice as she cried out "Gracias a Dios por ustedes!" (Thank God for you all!). It was in that moment, when I carried Gabriel's fragile body to his mother and sprawled him over her chest, that I realized how delicate life is. I remember gazing at the world around me and realizing that beyond language barriers, socioeconomic status, and cultural differences, we are all the same. Experiencing such profound satisfaction in helping those without the medical care they rightfully deserve inspired me to return with the appropriate medical training to further help those in need.

The miracle of medicine and the human body has never failed to astonish me. From a young age, I shadowed my father on his hospital rounds and imagined I was a health care provider as I scribbled in his patients' charts. I still have my life size anatomy and physiology coloring book that I would use to diagnose my imaginary patients. Although I admired my father's ability to manage his relentless health care service while providing his utmost support to his family, I dreamed of a profession that required less business management and focused more on patient care. Towards the end of my sophomore year of college, my father unexpectedly suffered from a stroke. My invincible hero now lay on a hospital bed, plugged into machines. I suddenly and painfully understood what it was like to be on the other side of the curtain. One night, as I sat bedside by my father, a physician assistant walked in to check on him. She asked a few questions and proceeded to check his heartbeat. She must have felt my worry since she looked at me and warmly asked, "Want to listen?" I had seen many physician assistants before that night, but this my first interaction with one. Meeting her that night, and witnessing the expertise and the compassion that she brought to her patients and their families, fueled my desire to become a PA.

I began to research the PA profession and developed relationships with a few who allowed me to shadow in different health care settings, such as nursing homes, hospitals, and clinics. Each impressed me with intelligence and empathy, always composed, yet able to work efficiently under pressure - qualities that I admire and patient care that I commend. They worked as a healthcare team, as opposed to the more independent healthcare I had witnessed most of my life. They comforted patients and thoroughly explained circumstances, as opposed to speaking in ambiguous medial terms. I continued working as a medical assistant at a healthcare clinic but lightened my load in my senior year, which I felt improved my academic performance. I found great reward in volunteering at the free Huda clinic in the underserved Detroit area. I worked mainly as a Spanish and Arabic translator, which inspired my medical aide trip to Caracas, Venezuela last summer. It was after my experience in South America that I felt a true calling to help those in particular who are less economically advantaged.

My father once told me, "You can be anything you want, as long as you put your mind to it." I am confident that I can and will achieve my goal of becoming an exceptional physician assistant. I look forward to the day when I hold the stethoscope up to a patient's ear and ask, "Want to listen?"

Essay 40 (539 words)

I have encountered many people and experiences in my life, but few have impressed upon me the deep desire and zeal to attend PA school like dancing with the Minnesota Ballet and teaching with Teach For America. These two very different yet definitive experiences changed and prepared me in profound ways.

While dancing for the Minnesota Ballet I was chosen to be the lead role in the Nutcracker. It was opening night and as I walked onto the stage feeling the warm lights and hearing the faint beginnings of the orchestra playing the first overture my mind turned off and the excitement and passion to perform took over. It wasn't until the standing ovation I reflected on all of the hard work and rehearsals that encompassed this profound and exciting experience. The Nutcracker performance was a moment I will never forget. In retrospect, I see the tremendous lessons I learned at an early age about passion and the incredible amount of hard work, discipline, teamwork, and enthusiasm it involved. Ballet was the first glimpse into my eventual pursuit into the PA profession.

Long after I set my ballet slippers aside I felt the familiar deep-rooted passion when I worked in a low-income middle school. I wrote the following in my journal half way through my Teach For America experience: "I am now two days over half way and realize the changes in who I am and in who my students are becoming. I visualize my student's faces, especially those moments that seem to be ingrained in my brain like a snapshot photograph. I see the face of one student as he admitted to me his involvement in gangs, the proud face of another student as he saw his 98% test score and even took it to the bathroom so no one could steal it. I see the tears in still another student's eyes because he's not at home caring for his mother, and the tears streaming down a mother's eyes as she pleads for any advice on how to raise her child." These are merely just a few of the moments that I realize have changed who I am. My Teach For America experience was much more profound than what I could've ever imagined. Each difficulty I persevered through I see myself as a more dedicated, passionate, and enthusiastic individual willing to serve despite the possibility of facing demanding circumstances. More so, I learned a new perspective, creativity, and desire to learn science and medicine through teaching others. I relished educating others about medicine and science yet I felt a strong desire to pursue a career that extended even further beyond the classroom.

I've learned the significance of working hard and persevering through tough circumstances for something I deeply desire. I have been strengthened and challenged through these experiences in what it means to not only be dedicated but also passionate. Subsequently, I discovered the PA profession encompasses the very things I had desired from my previous experiences. In my pursuit to attend PA school I anticipate the hard work, the challenge, and to face difficulties. I am confident I am fully prepared through what I've learned to carry each lesson forward with a fervor for medicine and a dedicated heart to serve.

Appendix

Special Guidelines for International Applicants

As has been mentioned, competition to get into a Physician Assistant program can be fierce. It can be even more difficult for international students since the application process requires more steps and can seem intimidating. However, many schools are interested in international students, so don't let the additional challenges discourage you.

There are a few things to consider though. You will need to be very well organized because there are multiple steps and deadlines to meet. Following these steps will help.

First, do a realistic assessment of your ability to do well in a program conducted entirely in English. You will be expected to read, write, and speak well in English. In addition to everyday language, you will need to be proficient in the knowledge of and use of medical terms. If your English is not what it needs to be, you will have problems. The best strategy then is to step back and work on your English skills before you apply to a program.

Once you are comfortable with your English, take the TOEFL (Test of English as a Foreign Language). Unless you have an undergraduate degree from an English-speaking university, the program will require you to take this test.

Third, assess your finances. In addition to the financial barriers facing any PA student, you will have additional expenses for travel—to and from school and if you go home during breaks. Be sure you can cover all your costs.

Fourth, gather your materials. Find out which transcripts are required by the program(s) to which you are applying and make sure you send everything in plenty of time to meet the deadlines. You will need to send transcripts from your other schools, so plan ahead for that as well.

Fifth, prepare for and take the GRE. Many graduate programs require this test. There are several ways to prepare ahead of time for the test, so take advantage of them and study for it.

Sixth, prepare for your visa application. You will want to apply for your visa as soon as you are accepted into a program, so know how to do that in advance of acceptance.

Finally, write, rewrite, and rewrite again your essay. If you are a nonnative English speaker, you will need assistance in writing the essay. Plan to spend plenty of time heeding the advice in this book. Also plan to get help from someone who can assist you with English.